# *Scope an*

## *for*

# *Nurse Administrators*

### *Second Edition*

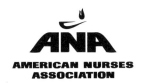

**AMERICAN NURSES
ASSOCIATION**

The Publishing Program of ANA

*Washington, D.C.*
*2004*

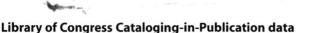

**Library of Congress Cataloging-in-Publication data**

American Nurses Association.
  Scope and standards for nurse administrators / American Nurses
Association.-- 2nd ed.
     p. ; cm.
Includes bibliographical references and index.
  ISBN 1-55810-217-5
  1.  Nursing services--Administration--Standards--United States. 2. Nurse
administrators--United States.
  [DNLM: 1.  Nursing Services--standards--United States. 2.  Nurse
Administrators--standards--United States. WY 100 A512sb 2003]  I. Title.

  RT89.A448 2003
  362.17'3'068--dc22
                                    2003023833

**Disclaimer:** The American Nurses Association (ANA) is a national professional association. This ANA publication—*Scope and Standards of Practice for Nurse Administrators, Second Edition*—reflects the thinking of the nursing profession on various issues and should be reviewed in conjunction with state board of nursing policies and practices. State law, rules, and regulations govern the practice of nursing, while *Scope and Standards of Practice for Nurse Administrators, Second Edition* guides nurses in the application of their professional skills and responsibilities.

Published by nursesbooks.org
The Publishing Program of ANA

American Nurses Association
600 Maryland Avenue, SW
Suite 100 West
Washington, DC 20024
1-800-274-4ANA
http://www.nursingworld.org/

ISBN 1-55810-217-5
03SSNA                           10M                          12/03

# Contents

# PREFACE

This document reflects the significant thinking, dialogue, and consensus decision-making of the American Nurses Association (ANA) specially convened expert workgroup composed of nurse administrators from diverse work and organizational settings. The nurse administrators included recognized leaders in the specialty. Each maintains membership in one or more specialty nursing organizations or other professional affiliations such as the American Organization of Nurse Executives (AONE), Association of State and Territorial Directors of Nursing (ASTDN), Hospice and Palliative Nurses Association (HPNA), and American Nurses Credentialing Center (ANCC) Magnet Recognition hospitals.

As part of the scope and standards development process, the workgroup examined previous versions of the ANA scope and standards of practice for nurse administrators (ANA, 1991, 1995), other associated standards documents (ANCC, 2003; ANA, 2004, 2000, 1996), and numerous contemporary and historical resources (AACN, 2002; AHCA, 2002; AHA, 2002, 2001; ANA, 2003, 2001, 1998; McClure & Langshawe, 2002; U.S. HHS, 2002). The 18-month process relied solely on telephone and electronic mail communication technologies. Upon completion of a draft document, the workgroup sought national and international comments during the field review period and posting at www.Nursingworld.org. This publication is the product of the workgroup's careful review and incorporation of those comments, review by the ANA Committee on Nursing Practice Standards and Guidelines, and final review and approval by the Congress on Nursing Practice and Economics.

## CONTRIBUTORS

### Workgroup:

Mary Etta Mills, ScD, RN, CNAA, FAAN, Chair
Barbara L. Baylis, MSN, RN, CPHQ
Doreen K. Frusti, MSN, MS, RN
Ada Sue Hinshaw, PhD, RN, FAAN
Patricia M. Kelley, RN, CHPN
Candia Baker Laughlin, MS,RN,C
Judy Lentz, RN, MSN, OCN, NHA
Joy F. Reed, EdD, RN
Karen Rush, BSN, BSW, CHPN
Jane Wall, RN, MSN, CNA

### ANA Staff

*Office of Nursing Practice & Policy*
Carol Bickford, PhD, RN
Mary Jean Schumann, MSN, RN, MBA CPNP
Yvonne Hulme, BBA

# STANDARDS FOR NURSE ADMINISTRATORS

## Standards of Practice

### STANDARD 1. ASSESSMENT
The nurse administrator develops, maintains, and evaluates patient and staff data collection systems and processes to support the practice of nursing and delivery of patient/client/resident care.

### STANDARD 2. PROBLEMS/DIAGNOSIS
The nurse administrator develops, maintains, and evaluates an environment that empowers and supports the professional nurse in analysis of assessment data and in decisions to determine relevant problems and diagnoses.

### STANDARD 3. IDENTIFICATION OF OUTCOMES
The nurse administrator develops, maintains, and evaluates information systems and processes that promote desired, patient/client/resident-defined, professional, and organizational outcomes.

### STANDARD 4. PLANNING
The nurse administrator develops, maintains, and evaluates organizational systems to facilitate planning for the delivery of care.

### STANDARD 5. IMPLEMENTATION
The nurse administrator develops, maintains, and evaluates organizational systems that support implementation of plans and delivery of care across the continuum.

### STANDARD 6. EVALUATION
The nurse administrator evaluates the plan and its progress in relation to the attainment of outcomes.

## Standards of Professional Performance

### STANDARD 7. QUALITY OF CARE AND ADMINISTRATIVE PRACTICE
The nurse administrator systematically evaluates the quality and effectiveness of nursing practice and nursing services administration.

### STANDARD 8. PERFORMANCE APPRAISAL
The nurse administrator evaluates personal performance based on professional practice standards, relevant statutes, rules and regulations, and organizational criteria.

### STANDARD 9. PROFESSIONAL KNOWLEDGE
The nurse administrator maintains and demonstrates current knowledge in the administration of healthcare organizations to advance nursing practice and the provision of quality healthcare services.

### STANDARD 10. PROFESSIONAL ENVIRONMENT
The nurse administrator is accountable for providing a professional environment.

### STANDARD 11. ETHICS
The nurse administrator's decisions and actions are based on ethical principles.

### STANDARDS 12. COLLABORATION
The nurse administrator collaborates with nursing staff at all levels, interdisciplinary teams, executive leaders, and other stakeholders.

### STANDARD 13. RESEARCH
The nurse administrator supports research and its integration into nursing and the delivery of healthcare services.

### STANDARD 14. RESOURCE UTILIZATION
The nurse administrator evaluates and administers the resources of nursing services.

# INTRODUCTION

Health care has always been a complex enterprise. Changing public expectations, regulations, resources, and service demands continue to challenge registered nurses and nurse administrators. Evolving technologies, reimbursement models, and consumer demands dictate shorter lengths of stay and other changes in treatment patterns. These issues, combined with an aging population, result in increasing patient acuity and larger volumes of patients moving from traditional acute care settings into ambulatory and long-term care environments. Nursing, itself composed of an aging workforce population, bears the brunt of such stressors throughout the healthcare delivery continuum.

The expectation for continuity of care across service delivery settings has gained momentum with consumers, payers, and providers as a means of increasing effectiveness and efficiency. Contracts, mergers, and partnerships are creating integrated delivery systems designed to foster coordination of care processes and services. This further emphasizes the need for nursing administration leadership capable of developing creative strategic plans to lead the healthcare system now and in the future. Innovative use of information technology, systems, and nursing research, and new fields of inquiry such as genetics and telehealth, offer opportunities to create practice environments not previously possible.

A time of great change and challenge is also a time of great opportunity for innovation. Legislative and regulatory constraints surround the management of human and material resources. As the demand for registered nurses intensifies and the supply declines, service-education partnerships offer increased strength in planning, marketing, educating, and mentoring a future nursing workforce. Nursing personnel and other healthcare discipline shortages also demand better explication and utilization of scopes of practice and interdisciplinary collaborative partnerships in delivering care and leading the organization. Increasing diversity of the patient population and the workforce makes it essential to support an inclusive environment and culture that creates synergy in systems and processes. These challenges further illustrate the interdependency of private and public health systems and complicate the role of the nurse administrator, thereby demanding skills in evaluation of complex systems and the development of collaborative solutions.

Systems-based issues abound. Concerns for confidentiality and security of patient health information have raised new legislative and technological issues in the transmission of information within and between healthcare settings and healthcare providers, including healthcare documentation access, monitoring, and interventions managed from a distance. Ethical considerations for new care opportunities offered by growth in clinical trial research and life-extending technological, genetic, and biologic interventions can generate multidisciplinary development of healthcare law and regulations, and related policies and procedures. The need for mass casualty readiness and emergency preparedness supports systems integration across the community of healthcare facilities, public health services, emergency response organizations, and government resources.

Also of concern are the continuing themes of resource allocation and revenue production that stem from increased competition, regulation, and cost while striving for excellence. These serve as an impetus for monitoring, evaluation, and performance improvement based on data that instructs both the business and practice of healthcare delivery. Effective and dynamic nurse administration leadership will ensure well-planned organizational structures, inclusive decision-making, creative and supportive personnel policies, professional models of care that promote excellent patient care services, collegial interdisciplinary relationships, and professional growth and development of nursing staff. The impact and effectiveness of such leadership will determine the future role of nursing in an evolving healthcare environment.

# Scope of Practice

The nurse administrator has most often been described as a registered nurse whose primary responsibility is the management of healthcare delivery services and who represents nursing services. Today's nurse administrator, however, is positioned at the vanguard of expanded roles and career opportunities resulting from a dynamic healthcare environment.

While traditional roles in all healthcare settings continue to offer career growth, new opportunities have also been created with the expansion of responsibilities for management of multiple patient/client/resident care services. At the corporate systems level of integrated care organizations, nurse administrators have opportunities to structure and plan nursing care systems across a continuum of services offered in multiple settings. These roles offer new challenges for nurse administrators to apply diverse skills in organizational analysis, strategic planning, financial and human resources management, and professional development.

Entrepreneurial opportunities have grown for nurse administrators interested in developing their own enterprises, such as community health services, assisted living, and adult day care. Expansion of clinical trials examining new therapeutic interventions has created a demand for individuals able to organize and manage complex regimens within and across research settings. Consultative roles require individuals prepared to apply advanced administrative knowledge and skill to settings that would benefit from new approaches to the management of healthcare services.

Diverse fields—such as quality of care evaluation, clinical and organizational ethics, information management, and legal and regulatory oversight—increasingly demand well-prepared nurse administrators. Often the nurse administrator is the sole healthcare professional as expanding career opportunities set the stage for a broad scope of nursing administration practice, evolving beyond the familiar hospital-based healthcare delivery model.

Nursing administration occurs in a wide variety of settings. These include small facilities, integrated delivery systems, larger corporate-owned facilities, and organizational and academic settings, as well as ambulatory and nontraditional environments. How nurse administrator positions are made operational will depend upon the structure and complexity of the settings in which they occur. Nevertheless, nurse administrators at all levels and in all types of settings share a common set of standards to guide practice in achieving their goals.

Whatever the venue, the nurse administrator has the responsibility to create a work environment that facilitates and encourages nursing staff to demonstrate accountability for their own practice, an environment that empowers registered nurses at all levels of the organization to utilize critical thinking and participate in decision-making that affects nursing practice. Creating such an environment requires openness to entrepreneurial partnerships, interdisciplinary collaboration, and leadership by all nurse administrators.

Therefore, communication is critical and mandates that structures and processes facilitate both vertical and horizontal communication. Productivity, quality of care, and a safe and healthy workplace are all enhanced when concern for the individual seeking healthcare services is the top priority and when nursing administrators assure:

- adequate numbers of clinically competent staff,
- positive working relationships among the healthcare team,
- autonomy and accountability for nursing practice,
- nursing control of nursing practice and the practice environment,
- adequate compensation commensurate with responsibilities, education, and experience,
- access to education and research,
- access to appropriate technologies, and
- promotion of evidence-based practice.

## Levels of Nursing Administration Practice

Nursing administration is conceptually divided into the administrative levels of the *nurse executive* and the *nurse manager*—each has a particular focus and makes a distinct contribution within a healthcare system. Some nurse administrator positions in diverse practice settings may contain components of more than one level. Individual nursing administrator positions may differ from the levels described in this scope of practice statement. However, most nursing administrative positions can be understood within this framework.

### Nurse Executive

The nurse executive is responsible and accountable for the overall management of nursing practice, nursing education and professional development, nursing research, nursing administration, and nursing services. The nurse executive holds the accountability to manage within the context of the organization as a whole, and to transform organizational values into daily operations yielding an efficient, effective, and caring organization. Such executive management responsibilities may by necessity be shared among many nurse administrators within the larger organization.

As the executive leader of a significant component of healthcare organization services and workforce, the nurse executive holds and exercises the authority to fulfill responsibilities to the profession, healthcare team, consumers of nursing services, and the organization. This authority is exercised globally across the organization's delivery systems and across the care continuum.

Serving as a catalyst and role model, the nurse executive provides leadership and direction in accord with the organization's mission and values and nursing's core ideology. The nurse executive collaborates with other professional disciplines to achieve organizational healthcare goals. The nurse executive is a partner with medicine, administrative executives, and other interdisciplinary organizational leaders to oversee practice and operations.

The nurse executive ensures the development, implementation, and evaluation of policies, programs, and services that are evidence-based and consistent with professional standards and values. The nurse executive is accountable for measurement, assessment, and improvement in nurse-sensitive patient and organizational outcomes, as well as the assurance of a professional nursing practice environment in which registered nurses are autonomous, govern their practice, and are empowered to provide effective, efficient, safe, and compassionate quality care. The practice environment is a critical factor in the recruitment and retention of registered nurses. The nurse executive is accountable to ensure the competence of registered nurses and their ongoing professional growth and development.

The nurse executive collaborates in the organization-wide healthcare delivery system and process design. Integral components of delivery system and process design include: the physical work environment (e.g., accommodating the aging worker), use of technology applications (i.e., more efficient, less personnel-intensive), nursing workload measurement based on patient need for nursing care, clinical and financial projection models, data collection and analysis, outcome identification and measurement, practice innovations, and recruitment and retention initiatives. Nurse executives provide leadership in professional, community, and legislative initiatives to shape the future of nursing, healthcare policy, and societal health.

The nurse executive addresses role accountabilities by collaborating with all relevant stakeholders to perform the following:

- Ensure that nursing practice is governed by professional nurses.

- Participate in the leadership of the healthcare organization as a full member of the executive team.

- Provide leadership in the strategic planning of the healthcare organization and nursing.

- Actively guide nursing as a profession to its objectives, such as those in *Nursing's Agenda for the Future* (ANA, 2002).

- Provide leadership in the determination of clinical, scholarly, and administrative nursing goals and directions, as well as the associated functions and processes necessary to achieve those goals.

- Acquire and allocate human, material, and financial resources for specific functions and processes.

- Evaluate and revise systems and processes of nursing services to ensure achievement of nurse-sensitive patient-, client-, or family-centered outcomes.

- Provide leadership in critical thinking, problem solving, managing conflict, and addressing ethical issues.

- Provide leadership in human resource development and management.

- Provide opportunities for consumer input into personal healthcare decisions and policy development.

- Ensure ongoing evaluation and innovation of services provided by nursing services and the organization as a whole.

- Facilitate the conduct, dissemination, and utilization of research to ensure evidence-based nursing, healthcare, management and administrative systems.

- Serve as a professional role model and mentor to motivate, develop, recruit, and retain future nurse administrators.

- Serve as an agent of change, assisting all staff in understanding the importance, necessity, impact, and process of change.

- Ensure that the diversity of the nursing workforce reflects population diversity.

- Ensure delivery of culturally-competent care.

- Support outcome measurement and evidence-based practice through participation in programs of study (e.g., National Database of Nursing Quality Indicators).

- Ensure measurement of patient/client/resident need for nursing care and then allocate resources accordingly.

- Ensure registered nurse participation in decision-making at varied levels of the organization.

- Ensure integration of appropriate technologies to meet the needs of professional nursing.

- Ensure a safe working environment.

- Strive to meet the Nursing Advisory Council on Nurse Education and Practice (NACNEP) goal of two-thirds of the registered nurse workforce prepared at the baccalaureate degree in nursing or higher education level by 2010.

In today's continuously evolving health care environment and delivery system models, the nurse executive may be identified by other titles such as the Chief Nursing Officer (CNO), Senior Vice President, Director of Clinical Nursing Services, Vice President for Patient Services, Service Chief, Chief Executive Officer, Chief Operating Officer, Director, President, Dean, or Associate Dean.


### Nurse Manager

Nurse managers are responsible to a nurse executive and manage one or more defined areas of nursing services. Nurse managers advocate for and allocate available resources to promote efficient, effective, safe, and compassionate nursing care based on current standards of practice. They promote shared decision-making and professional autonomy by providing input—their own and that of their staff—into executive-level decisions, and by keeping staff informed of executive level activities and vice versa. Other responsibilities vary depending on the size and function of the organization.

Nurse managers coordinate activities between defined areas, and provide clinical and administrative leadership and expertise. They facilitate an atmosphere of interactive management and the development of collegial relationships among nursing personnel and others. They serve as a link between nursing personnel and other healthcare disciplines and workers throughout the organization and within the healthcare community. Nurse managers have major responsibility for the implementation of the vision, mission, philosophy, core values, evidence-based practice, and standards of the organization, and nursing services within their defined areas of responsibility.

Nurse managers are accountable for the environment in which clinical nursing is practiced. The nurse manager must create a learning environment that is open and respectful, and promotes the sharing of expertise to promote the benefits of health outcomes. The ability of nurse managers to enhance the practice environment is critical to the recruitment and retention of registered nurses with diverse backgrounds and appropriate education and experience. Nurse managers contribute to the strategic planning process, day-to-day operations, standards of care, and attainment of goals of the organization. Nurse managers collaborate with the nurse executive and others in organizational planning, innovation, and evaluation. In larger organizations, the nurse manager may include further delineated levels.

To fulfill the responsibilities described above, the nurse manager, in collaboration with nursing personnel and members of other disciplines, performs the following:

- Ensure that care is delivered with respect for individuals' rights and preferences.
- Participate in nursing and organizational policy formulation and decision-making involving staff.
- Accept organizational accountability for services provided to recipients.
- Evaluate the quality and appropriateness of health care.
- Coordinate nursing care with other healthcare disciplines, and assist in integrating services across the continuum of health care.
- Participate in the recruitment, selection, and retention of personnel, including staff representative of the population diversity.
- Assess the impact of, and plan strategies to address, such issues as:
    - Ethnic, cultural and diversity changes in the population
    - Political and social influences
    - Financial and economic issues
    - The aging of society and demographic trends
    - Ethical issues related to health care

- Assume responsibility for staffing and scheduling personnel. Assignments reflect appropriate utilization of personnel, considering scope of practice, competencies, patient/client/resident needs, and complexity of care.
- Ensure appropriate orientation, education, credentialing, and continuing professional development for personnel.
- Provide guidance for and supervision of personnel accountable to the nurse manager.
- Evaluate performance of personnel.
- Develop, implement, monitor, and be accountable for the budget for the defined area(s) of responsibility.
- Ensure evidence-based practice by participating in and involving the nursing staff in evaluative research activities.
- Provide or facilitate educational experiences for nursing and other students.
- Ensure shared accountability for professional practice.
- Advocate for a work environment that minimizes work-related illness and injury.

Like the nurse executive level, nurse administrators at the manager level may be identified by other titles, such as District Supervisor, Head Nurse, Department Head, Shift Manager, Clinical Coordinator, Project Manager, or Division Officer.

## Qualifications of Nurse Administrators

Given the expectations of leadership and accountability of the nurse administrator, it is important to define the licensure, education, and experience required. Both the nurse executive and the nurse manager must hold an active registered nurse license and meet the requirements in the state in which they practice.

The nurse executive should hold a bachelor's degree and master's degree with a major in nursing. A doctoral degree in a relevant field is recommended, as is a nationally recognized certification in nursing administration.

The nurse manager should be prepared with a minimum of a bachelor's degree with a major in nursing. A master's degree with a focus in nursing is recommended, as is nationally recognized certification in nursing administration and an appropriate specialty.

The experience backgrounds of professional nurses who serve as nurse administrators must include clinical and administrative practice, which enables these registered nurses to consistently fulfill the responsibilities inherent in their respective administrative roles. The nurse administrator's practice draws on knowledge and research from such areas as noted in Table 1:

*Table 1. Knowledge Base of Nurse Administrator Practice*

| | |
|---|---|
| • Care management systems | • Negotiation and conflict resolution |
| • Clinical practice guidelines and best practices | • Nursing research and other scholarly activities |
| • Consumer healthcare issues | • Organizational behavior and development |
| • Customer service | |
| • Data management | • Patient and employee safety regulations |
| • Evidence-based nursing administration | • Performance improvement |
| • Fiscal management and financial outcome | • Practice innovation |
| • Health and public policy | • Professional nursing practice |
| • Healthcare economics | • Professional practice environment |
| • Healthcare evaluation and outcome measures | • Standards of clinical nursing practice |
| • Law, regulation, and ethics | • Strategic visioning and planning |
| • Management systems, processes, and analysis | • Systems for patient safety |
| • Marketing initiatives | • Technologies |
| • Measurement of patient needs, outcomes, nursing workload | • Trends in business practices |
| *Adapted from (VHA, 2000).* | |

## Summary of Nurse Executive and Nurse Manager

Table 2 compares the nurse administrator levels of nurse executive and nurse manager. Although some holding these positions have yet to complete the recommended educational and certification qualifications, this publication encourages all nurse administrators to achieve these professional milestones.

**Table 2. Comparison of Qualifications and Responsibilities for Nurse Executive and Nurse Manager**

| Item | Nurse Executive | Nurse Manager |
|---|---|---|
| License | In state of practice | In state of practice |
| Education | BS, MS with focus in nursing Doctorate recommended | BS with focus in nursing MS with focus in nursing recommended |
| Certification | Nursing Administration recommended | Nursing Administration and appropriate specialty recommended |
| Authority | Organization-wide | One or more assigned areas |
| Area(s) of responsibility | Whole organization | Assigned areas only |
| Fiduciary responsibility | Input into system-wide budget planning  Clinical/financial projections and budget for entire nursing department | Budget for assigned areas only |
| Specific responsibilities | Partner with other disciplinesand leaders  Acquires resources for function and process  Ensures development of policies, programs, and evidence-based practice consistent with standards  Leads and directs patient care delivery systems  Provides leadership in human resources development and management  Visionary, strategic planner, change agent, practice innovator  Accountable for continuous quality improvement for entire nursing system  Assures nurse participation in decision-making | Direct supervision of assigned staff and interdisciplinary collaboration  Manages recruitment, selection, retention, staffing, scheduling, and assigning  Empowers staff to develop policies with management oversight  Accepts organizational accountability for services provided  Directs and manages personnel for assigned areas  Implements the vision, mission, philosophy, core values, evidence-based practice, and standards in assigned areas  Evaluates quality and appropriateness of healthcare delivery for assigned areas  Empowers staff to participate in decision-making |

# STANDARDS OF PRACTICE
# AND
# PROFESSIONAL PERFORMANCE

Standards are authoritative statements by which the nursing profession describes the responsibilities for which its practitioners are accountable. Consequently, standards reflect the values and priorities of the profession. Standards provide direction for professional nursing practice and a framework for the evaluation of this practice. Written in measurable terms, standards also define the nursing profession's accountability to the public and the outcomes for which registered nurses are responsible.

Specific measurement criteria accompany each of the standards of practice and professional performance for nurse administrators. At this time, research and the existing body of knowledge have not identified measurement criteria specific to either the nurse executive or nurse manager levels. Because the focus of this specialty practice tends to be on the development, implementation, and evaluation of the supporting framework, processes, and environment of nursing practice, the language of some of the standards and measurement criteria have been modified from those referenced in *Standards of Clinical Nursing Practice, 2nd Edition* (ANA, 1998). For example, the Standards of Practice describe the nursing process in nursing administration as assessment, problem/diagnosis, identification of outcomes, planning, implementation, and evaluation.

# STANDARDS OF PRACTICE

## STANDARD 1. ASSESSMENT

**The nurse administrator develops, maintains, and evaluates patient/ client/resident and staff data collection systems and processes to support the practice of nursing and delivery of patient/client/resident care.**

*Measurement Criteria*

The nurse administrator:

1. Identifies assessment elements specific to nursing patient/client/resident indicators appropriate to a given organization.

2. Utilizes current research findings and current practice guidelines and standards to modify and improve data collection elements.

3. Monitors and evaluates assessment processes that are sensitive to the unique and diverse needs of individuals and target populations.

4. Identifies and documents the necessary resources to support data collection, and secures appropriate resources.

5. Analyzes the workflow related to effectiveness and efficiency of assessment processes.

6. Provides for efficient data collection as part of the institutional data collection systems.

7. Promotes, maintains, and evaluates a data collection system that has an accessible and retrievable format.

8. Initiates mechanisms to modify information systems and processes as needed to meet changing data requirements and needs.

9. Collaborates with appropriate departments to utilize assessment data to improve the operation of the healthcare environment and facility.

10. Evaluates assessment practices to assure timely, reliable, valid, and comprehensive data collection.

11. Facilitates integration of uniform assessment processes developed in collaboration with other healthcare disciplines across the continuum of care and internal and external to the organization.

12. Develops criteria and establishes procedures to assure confidentiality of data.

## STANDARD 2. PROBLEMS/DIAGNOSIS

**The nurse administrator develops, maintains, and evaluates an environment that empowers and supports the professional nurse in analysis of assessment data and in decisions to determine relevant problems and diagnoses.**

*Measurement Criteria*

The nurse administrator:

1. Identifies and secures adequate resources for decision analysis in collaboration with appropriate departments.

2. Assists and supports staff in developing and maintaining problem/diagnosis competency.

3. Facilitates interdisciplinary collaboration in data analysis and decision-making process.

4. Promotes an organizational climate that supports validation of problems/diagnoses.

5. Assures a system of documentation of problems/diagnoses that facilitates development of a patient/client/resident-centered plan of care and determination of desired outcomes.

6. Formulates a diagnosis of the organization's environment, culture, and priorities that direct and support care delivery.

## Standard 3. Identification of Outcomes

**The nurse administrator develops, maintains, and evaluates information systems and processes that promote desired, patient/client/resident-defined, professional, and organizational outcomes.**

*Measurement Criteria*

The nurse administrator:

1. Participates in the design and development of interdisciplinary processes to establish and maintain standards consistent with the identified outcomes.

2. Facilitates participation of registered nurses, other staff members, and patients/clients/residents in interdisciplinary identification of desired outcomes.

3. Assists in identification, development, and utilization of databases that include nursing measures and desired outcomes.

4. Facilitates registered nurse participation in the monitoring and evaluation of nursing care in accordance with established professional, regulatory, and organizational standards of practice.

5. Fosters establishment and continuous improvement of clinical guidelines related to outcomes that provide direction for continuity of care and that are attainable with available resources.

6. Collaborates with appropriate departments in the development of integrated systems to support nursing service delivery.

7. Promotes the integration of clinical, human resource, and financial data to support decision-making.

## STANDARD 4. PLANNING

**The nurse administrator develops, maintains, and evaluates organizational systems to facilitate planning for the delivery of care.**

*Measurement Criteria*

The nurse administrator:

1.  Facilitates the development and continuous improvement of organizational systems in which plans related to the delivery of nursing services can be developed, modified, documented, and evaluated.

2.  Facilitates the development and continuous improvement of organizational systems that promote plans and support the prioritization of activities related to patient/client/resident-directed care and the delivery of nursing services.

3.  Facilitates the development and continuous improvement of mechanisms for plans to be recorded, reviewed, and updated across the continuum of care.

4.  Promotes organizational processes that allow for creativity in the development of alternative plans for achieving desired, patient/client/resident-defined, cost-effective outcomes.

5.  Fosters interdisciplinary planning and collaboration that focuses on the individuals and populations served.

6.  Promotes the integration of applicable contemporary management and organizational theories, nursing and related research findings, and practice standards and guidelines into the planning process.

7.  Assists and supports staff in developing and maintaining competency in the planning and change process.

8.  Advocates for integration of policies into action plans for achieving desired outcomes.

9.  Participates in the development, implementation, and use of a system to promote the rights and ethical treatment of the patient/client/resident and to ensure that abuse of the patient/client/resident's rights is reported.

10. Reviews and evaluates plans for appropriate utilization of staff at all levels of practice in accordance with the provisions of the state's nurse practice act and the professional standards of practice.

11. Integrates clinical, human resource, and financial data to appropriately plan nursing and patient/client/resident care across a continuum.

12. Collaborates with appropriate departments and disciplines for the entire system to operate more efficiently in achieving outcomes.

13. Advocates for staff involvement in all levels of organizational planning and decision-making.

## STANDARD 5. IMPLEMENTATION

**The nurse administrator develops, maintains, and evaluates organizational systems that support implementation of plans and delivery of care across the continuum.**

*Measurement Criteria*

The nurse administrator:

1. Participates in the development, evaluation, and maintenance of organizational systems that integrate policies and procedures with regulations, practice standards, and clinical guidelines.

2. Designs and improves systems and identifies resources that support interventions that are consistent with the established plans.

3. Facilitates staff participation in decision-making regarding the development and implementation of organizational systems, and the specification of resources necessary for implementation of the plan.

4. Collaborates in the design and improvement of systems and the identification of resources that assure interventions are safe, effective, efficient, age-relevant, and culturally sensitive.

5. Collaborates in the design and improvement of systems and processes that assure interventions are implemented by the appropriate personnel.

6. Collaborates in the design and improvement of systems to assure appropriate and efficient documentation of interventions and patient/client/resident responses.

7. Leads initiatives in innovative programs and new implementation alternatives.

## Standard 6. Evaluation

**The nurse administrator evaluates the plan and its progress in relation to the attainment of outcomes.**

*Measurement Criteria*

The nurse administrator:

1. Promotes implementation of processes that deliver data and information to empower staff in decision-making.

2. Ensures educational opportunities for staff based on evaluation findings—specific to the population served, professional practice, available technologies, or required skills—to enhance quality in health care delivery.

3. Utilizes appropriate research methods and findings to evaluate and improve care processes, structures, and measurement of desired outcomes.

4. Facilitates the participation of staff in the systematic, interdisciplinary, and ongoing evaluation of programs, processes, and desired outcomes that promote organizational effectiveness.

5. Sets priorities for allocation of resources to conduct evaluative activities.

6. Ensures sufficient resources to provide for the critical assessment and evaluation of desired outcomes, including allocation of individual staff time for meaningful involvement.

7. Fosters participation and recognition of staff in internal and external, formal and informal organizational evaluation committees, teams, and task forces.

8. Advocates for and supports a process of participative decision-making.

9. Participates in the evaluation of all appropriate healthcare providers through privileging, credentialing, or certification processes.

10. Supports information handling processes and technologies to facilitate evaluation of effectiveness and efficiency of decisions, plans, and activities in relation to desired outcomes.

11. Promotes the development of policies, procedures, and guidelines based on research findings and institutional measurement of quality outcomes.

12. Utilizes data generated from outcomes research to develop innovative changes in care delivery.

# Standards of Professional Performance

## Standard 7. Quality of Care and Administrative Practice

**The nurse administrator systematically evaluates the quality and effectiveness of nursing practice and nursing services administration.**

*Measurement Criteria*

*The nurse administrator:*

1. Leads the development, implementation, and improvement of care delivery models and services that meet or exceed customer expectations.

2. Identifies key indicators including measures of quality, safety, other outcomes of nursing practice, and customer needs and expectations.

3. Advocates for and participates in the development of clinical, operational, and financial processes from which key outcomes indicators can be derived, reported, and used for improvement.

4. Leads in creating and evaluating systems, processes and programs that support organizational and nursing core values and objectives.

5. Evaluates the care environment to ensure that it is safe and healthful for patients/client/resident and staff.

6. Implements performance improvement measures for the key indicators that have been identified.

## STANDARD 8. PERFORMANCE APPRAISAL

**The nurse administrator evaluates personal performance based on professional practice standards, relevant statutes, rules and regulations, and organizational criteria.**

*Measurement Criteria*

*The nurse administrator:*

1. Identifies industry trends and competencies in nursing administration and nursing practice, using a systematic process.

2. Engages in self-assessment of role accountabilities on a regular basis, identifying areas of strength as well as areas for professional and practice development.

3. Evaluates accomplishment of the strategic plan and the vision for professional nursing.

4. Seeks constructive feedback regarding one's own practice.

5. Takes action to achieve plans for performance improvement.

6. Participates in peer review as appropriate.

## Standard 9. Professional Knowledge

**The nurse administrator maintains and demonstrates current knowledge in the administration of healthcare organizations to advance nursing practice and the provision of quality healthcare services.**

*Measurement Criteria*

The nurse administrator:

1. Seeks experiences to advance one's skills and knowledge base in areas of responsibilities including the art and science of nursing, changes in healthcare systems, application of emerging technologies, and administrative practices.

2. Demonstrates a commitment to lifelong learning and ongoing professional development through such activities as education, certification, and participation in professional organizations.

3. Networks with state, regional, national, and global peers to share ideas and conduct mutual problem solving.

## STANDARD 10. PROFESSIONAL ENVIRONMENT

**The nurse administrator is accountable for providing a professional environment.**

*Measurement Criteria*

*The nurse administrator:*

1.  Creates a professional practice environment that fosters excellence in nursing services.

2.  Creates a climate of effective communication.

3.  Fosters empowered decision-making, accountability, and autonomy in nursing practice for professional nurses.

4.  Leads the organization of nursing services through a well-established nursing leadership structure, and is a formal authority participant in organizational leadership.

5.  Establishes and promotes a framework for professional nursing practice built on core ideology which includes vision, mission, philosophy, core values, evidence-based practice, and standards of practice.

6.  Assures the work environment is one of mutual respect for the individual and the profession.

7.  Develops strategies to recruit and retain, mentor, assure quality education and training, and ensure meaningful work to maximize job satisfaction and professional development of nursing staff.

8.  Promotes understanding and effective use of organization, management, and nursing theories and research.

9.  Actively participates in the general and nursing management education and professional development of staff, students, and colleagues.

10. Advocates for organizational adherence to the ANA *Bill of Rights for Registered Nurses* (ANA, 2001a).

11. Shares knowledge and skills with students, colleagues and others, and acts as a role model and mentor.

## Standard 11. Ethics

**The nurse administrator's decisions and actions are based on ethical principles.**

*Measurement Criteria*

*The nurse administrator:*

1. Advocates on behalf of recipients of services and personnel.

2. Maintains privacy, confidentiality, and security of patient/client/resident, staff, and organization data.

3. Adheres to the *Code of Ethics for Nurses with Interpretive Statements* (ANA, 2001b).

4. Assures compliance with regulatory and professional standards, as well as integrity in business practices.

5. Fosters a nondiscriminatory climate in which care is delivered in a manner sensitive to sociocultural diversity.

6. Assures a process to identify and address ethical issues within nursing and the organization.

## STANDARDS **12.** COLLABORATION

**The nurse administrator collaborates with nursing staff at all levels, interdisciplinary teams, executive leaders, and other stakeholders.**

*Measurement Criteria*

*The nurse administrator:*

1.  Facilitates and models collaboration within nursing services, the organization, and the community.

2.  Collaborates with nursing staff and other disciplines at all levels in the development, implementation, and evaluation of programs and services.

3.  Collaborates with administrative peers in determining the acquisition, allocation, and utilization of fiscal and human resources.

4.  Develops and fosters relationships that support the continuous enhancement of care delivery and patient/client/resident and employee satisfaction.

## STANDARD 13. RESEARCH

**The nurse administrator supports research and its integration into nursing and the delivery of healthcare services.**

*Measurement Criteria*

*The nurse administrator:*

1. Creates the environment and advocates for resources supportive of nursing research and scholarly inquiry.

2. Assures nursing research priorities align with nursing's and the organization's strategic plan and objectives.

3. Supports research that promotes evidence-based, clinically effective and efficient, nurse-sensitive patient/client/resident outcomes and other healthcare outcomes.

4. Facilitates the dissemination of research findings and the integration of evidence-based guidelines and practices into health care.

5. Supports procedures for review of proposed research studies, including protection of the rights of human subjects.

6. Identifies areas of clinical and administrative inquiry suitable for nurse researchers.

## STANDARD 14. RESOURCE UTILIZATION

**The nurse administrator evaluates and administers the resources of nursing services.**

*Measurement Criteria*

*The nurse administrator:*

1. Assures nursing workload is measured and resources are allocated based upon patient/client/resident need.

2. Develops systems to continuously monitor and measure the quality, safety, and outcomes of nursing services.

3. Develops, values, and expands the intellectual capital of the organization.

4. Assures and optimizes fiscal resource allocation to support current and potential nursing objectives and initiatives.

5. Provides fiscal oversight of allocated resources to optimize the provision of quality, cost-effective care.

6. Guides the delegation of responsibilities appropriate to the credentialing, education, and experience of staff.

7. Designs and negotiates organizational acceptance of appropriate roles for the utilization of all staff.

8. Monitors and evaluates appropriate utilization of staff.

9. Leads in promoting the appropriate use of innovative applications and new technologies throughout the continuum of care.

# Glossary

**Continuity of care.** An interdisciplinary process that includes patients and significant others in the development and implementation of a plan of coordinated care. This process facilitates the transition of a patient/client/resident between settings and services, based on changing needs and available resources.

**Core ideology.** Vision, mission, philosophy, core values, evidence-based practice, and standards of practice.

**Criteria.** Relevant, measurable indicators of the standards of practice and professional performance.

**Data collection systems and processes.** Mechanisms and tools to identify and gather the necessary measures and information used in analysis, decision-making, action, and evaluation.

**Evidence-based practice.** A process based on the collection, interpretation, and integration of valid, important, and applicable data, information, and knowledge preferably derived from research findings to define the best approach or solution.

**Healthcare organization.** The total healthcare entity within which nursing services operate.

**Intellectual capital.** An organization's valued human knowledge, professional skills, applied experience, organizational technology, and customer relationships that provide its competitive edge in the industry or market.

**Nurse administrator.** A registered nurse whose primary responsibility is the management of healthcare services delivery, and who represents nursing services. For purposes of this document, the two levels of nurse administrators are those of the nurse executive and the nurse manager.

**Nurse executive.** A registered nurse who is accountable for nursing services, and manages from the perspective of the organization as a whole.

**Nurse manager.** A registered nurse who manages one or more defined areas within nursing services.

**Nurse-sensitive.** Reflective of the impact of nursing actions on patient/client/resident outcomes.

**Nursing services.** The structure through which services, including direct care, education, or any other nursing related services, are provided by registered nurses and other personnel under the direction of a nurse administrator, within the scope of nursing practice, and in accordance with state laws and regulations.

**Patient/client/resident.** An individual, family, group, community, or population receiving care provided by nursing services.

**Staff.** All personnel reporting to the nurse administrator.

**Standard.** An authoritative statement defined, recognized, and published by the profession and by which the quality of practice, service, or education can be judged.

**Standards of practice.** Authoritative statements that describe a competent level of practice demonstrated through assessment, diagnosis and problem identification, identification of outcomes, planning, implementation, and evaluation.

**Standards of professional performance.** Authoritative statements that describe a competent level of behavior in the professional role, including activities related to quality of care and administrative practice, performance appraisal, education, professional environment, ethics, collaboration, research, and resource utilization.

# REFERENCES

American Association of Colleges of Nursing (2002). *Hallmarks of the professional nursing practice environment*, January. Washington, DC: AACN.

American Health Care Association (2002). *Competencies for senior nurse leaders in LTC vision statement. Washington, DC: AHCA.*

American Hospital Association (2001). *Workforce supply for hospitals and health systems: Issues and recommendations.* Washington, DC: AHA.

American Nurses Association. (2004). *Nursing: Scope and standards of practice.* Washington, DC: Nursesbooks.org.

American Hospital Association (2002). *In our hands: How hospital leaders can build a thriving workforce.* April. Chicago: AHA.

American Nurses Association. (2003). *Nursing's social policy statement, Second edition.* Washington, DC: Nursesbooks.org.

American Nurses Association (2002). *Nursing's agenda for the future: A call to the nation.* Washington, DC: ANA.

American Nurses Association (2001a). *Bill of rights for registered nurses.* Washington, DC: ANA.

American Nurses Association (2001b). *Code of ethics for nursing with interpretive statements.* Washington, DC: American Nurses Publishing.

American Nurses Association (2000). *Scope and standards of practice for nursing professional development.* Washington, DC: American Nurses Publishing.

American Nurses Association (1998). *Standards of clinical nursing practice, 2nd edition.* Washington, DC: American Nurses Publishing.

American Nurses Association. (1996). *Scope and standards of advanced practice registered nursing.* Washington, DC: American Nurses Publishing.

American Nurses Association (1995). *Scope and standards for nurse administrators.* Washington, DC: American Nurses Publishing.

American Nurses Association (1991). *Standards for organized nursing services and responsibilities of nurse administrators across all settings.* Kansas City, MO: ANA.

American Nurses Credentialing Center 2003. *Magnet Recognition Program instruction and application process manual (2003–2004).* Washington, DC: ANCC.

McClure, M. & Hinshaw, A. S. (2002). *Magnet hospitals revisited: Attraction and retention of professional nurses.* Washington, DC: American Nurses Publishing.

VHA. National Nursing Leadership Council (2000). *Revolutionizing the future of nursing care: Defining the role of the chief nursing officer in the 21st century.* Irving, TX: VHA.

U.S. Department of Health and Human Services (2002). *The registered nurse population: Findings from the National Sample Survey of Registered Nurses, March 2000.* Washington, DC: Health Resources and Services Administration, Bureau of Health Professions, Division of Nursing.

# APPENDIX A
## ANA *Bill of Rights for Registered Nurses* (2001)

Registered nurses promote and restore health, prevent illness, and protect the people entrusted to their care. They work to alleviate the suffering experienced by individuals, families, groups, and communities. In so doing, nurses provide services that maintain respect for human dignity and embrace the uniqueness of each patient and the nature of his or her health problems, without restriction with regard to social or economic status. To maximize the contributions nurses make to society, it is necessary to protect the dignity and autonomy of nurses in the workplace. To that end, the following rights must be afforded:

1. Nurses have the right to practice in a manner that fulfills their obligations to society and to those who receive nursing care.

2. Nurses have the right to practice in environments that allow them to act in accordance with professional standards and legally authorized scopes of practice.

3. Nurses have the right to a work environment that supports and facilitates ethical practice, in accordance with the *Code of Ethics for Nurses with Interpretive Statements*.

4. Nurses have the right to freely and openly advocate for themselves and their patients, without fear of retribution.

5. Nurses have the right to fair compensation for their work, consistent with their knowledge, experience, and professional responsibilities.

6. Nurses have the right to a work environment that is safe for themselves and for their patients.

7. Nurses have the right to negotiate the conditions of their employment, either as individuals or collectively, in all practice settings.

Adopted by the ANA, Board of Directors, June 26, 2001.

# APPENDIX B
## *Standards for Organized Services* (1991)

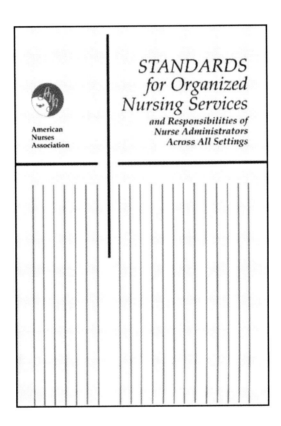

# CONTENTS

# INTRODUCTION

Dramatic, sweeping changes will continue to influence the process and focus of health care delivery. Social changes, regulatory and organizational changes, and changes in the approach to nursing management are widespread and affect nurses across all health care settings. Legislation has been enacted that increases both governmental and consumer involvement in making health care decisions. Social and demographic changes include sharp increases in the number of older persons, the number of women working outside the home, and the number of single-parent families.

More older persons need assistance with the activities of daily living than before, but fewer family members are available to provide that support. There is a new focus on legal and ethical issues and greater attention to individual rights. The Medicare prospective payment system, legislated in 1981 and implemented in 1983, has given impetus to the development of alternative delivery systems and the increased use of community-based health care. Technological advances have created both an educational need among health care providers and ethical and human relations concerns for providers and the public. All of these changes have brought challenges and new opportunities to nurse administrators wherever nursing services are provided.

The primary goal of organized nursing services is the delivery of effective nursing care to individuals. To meet the new demands placed on organized nursing services, nurse administrators must be knowledgeable, skilled, and competent in directing clinical practice, in data analysis, in business management, and in resource management. Nurse administrators are responsible for the provision of safe, efficient, cost-effective care to recipients served by organized nursing services.

The scope and responsibilities of the nurse administrator are increasing across all health care settings. The nurse executive frequently has corporate responsibilities, as is the case in multisystem chains. The nurse executive may be the entrepreneur and/or the chief executive officer, as is frequently the case in nursing centers, home care agencies, and other settings. Within the organization, the responsibilities of the nurse executive have been expanded horizontally to include areas outside nursing. At times, organized nursing services have been expanded to include additional services provided by satellite units.

Expenditures for nursing services are rising because of expenditures to recruit and retain nurses, an increase in patient acuity, and competition for nurses. There are also reports of increased revenue generated by organized nursing services.[1]

To provide guidance to nurse administrators in addressing recent changes in the health care environment, the American Nurses Association (ANA) has revised two ANA publications: *Standards for Organized Nursing Services* (1982) and *Roles, Responsibilities, and Qualifications for Nurse Administrators* (1978).[2,3] ANA thanks the organizations that were represented on the task force that developed this document: the American Health Care Association, the American Organization of Nurse Executives, the Association of Directors of Nursing in Long-Term Care, the National Association for Home Care, and the National Gerontological Nursing Association.

The standards presented herein apply to all settings in which nursing services are delivered, including hospitals, long-term facilities, community health centers, home health agencies, and nursing centers.

The responsibilities and qualifications of nurse administrators are defined, with distinctions drawn between the nurse executive and nurse manager. The Appendix provides a comparison of the roles of nurse executive and nurse manager. The Glossary gives definitions for *defined area, health care organization, nurse administrator* (with the two levels of nursing administration being those of the nurse executive and the nurse manager), *organized nursing services, recipient of care,* and *standard.*

# STANDARDS FOR ORGANIZED NURSING SERVICES

## Standard I. Philosophy and Structure

ORGANIZED NURSING SERVICES HAVE A PHILOSOPHY AND STRUCTURE THAT ENSURE THE DELIVERY OF EFFECTIVE NURSING CARE.

*Rationale*

The philosophy provides the statement of beliefs and values that gives direction to the delivery of nursing services. The structure of organized nursing services is developed to make the philosophy operational. It is necessary to have a philosophy and structure to ensure a framework for the provision of nursing care and to provide a means for resolving nursing practice problems.

*Criteria*

1. The philosophy and structure are compatible with established professional standards, *Nursing: A Social Policy Statement* and *Code for Nurses with Interpretive Statements*, standards of regulatory agencies, and the mission of the organization within which nursing services are provided. [4,5,6]

2. The philosophy of organized nursing services provides to individual nurses the authority and accountability for the clinical management of nursing practice.

3. The philosophy provides for a structure that facilitates participative management.

4. A written organizational plan specifies lines of authority, accountability, and responsibility for all nursing personnel.

5. The philosophy supports the representation and participation of nurses in professional organizations and community and governmental activities related to health care.

## Standard II. Nurse Administrator

ORGANIZED NURSING SERVICES ARE ADMINISTERED BY
QUALIFIED AND COMPETENT NURSE ADMINISTRATORS.

*Rationale*

The complex demands of the health care environment require
the leadership and direction of qualified and competent nurse administrators (nurse executives and nurse managers) for the provision of effective nursing care.*

*Criteria*

1. The nurse executive is a registered nurse who holds a baccalaureate degree in nursing and a graduate degree in nursing or a related field from a program that includes organizational science and management concepts. Certification in
   nursing administration by a nationally recognized nursing
   organization is recommended.

2. The nurse manager is a registered nurse prepared with a
   minimum of a baccalaureate degree in nursing. A graduate
   degree in nursing or a related field is recommended, as is
   certification in nursing administration by a nationally recognized nursing organization.

3. Nurse administrators maintain knowledge of current technology and trends in health care.

4. Nurse administrators collaborate with nursing staff at all
   levels in the development, implementation, and evaluation
   of programs within organized nursing services.

5. Nurse administrators establish and maintain formal and informal relationships within the organization which facilitate
   goal attainment for organized nursing services.

6. The nurse executive is a member of the policy-making body

---

*A complete description of the levels, responsibilities, and qualifications of nurse
administrators is presented in the next section of this publication.

of the organization.

7. Nurse administrators represent organized nursing services within decision-making bodies in the organization.

8. Nurse administrators advocate for the nurses they manage, as well as for the recipients of nursing care.

## Standard III. Fiscal Resource Management

THE NURSE EXECUTIVE DETERMINES AND ADMINISTERS THE FISCAL RESOURCES OF ORGANIZED NURSING SERVICES. THE NURSE EXECUTIVE HAS AN INTERACTIVE ROLE IN THE DETERMINATION OF THE ORGANIZATION'S FISCAL RESOURCE REQUIREMENTS AND THEIR ACQUI-SITION, ALLOCATION, AND UTILIZATION.

*Rationale*

Organized nursing services must be administered by an executive aware of nursing's contribution to the overall resource framework of the organization. This requires the nurse executive to be accountable for and have commensurate authority for determination of resources. In some settings, the nurse executive delegates to nurse managers responsibility for fiscal resource management of defined areas. Accountability for the budget of organized nursing services as a whole remains with the nurse executive.

*Criteria*

1. The budget for organized nursing services is developed by the nurse executive and nurse managers for designated areas; the budget is generated and controlled by the nurse executive with input from nurse managers.

2. Organized nursing services identify, implement, and maximize current and potential sources of organizational revenue generated by nursing activities.

3. The nurse executive collaborates with the chief executive officer and other executives of the organization in determining the acquisition, allocation, and utilization of the organization's fiscal resources.

4. Organized nursing services have a financial information system that provides data needed to monitor and explain variances from established budgetary parameters.

## Standard IV. Nursing Process

WITHIN ORGANIZED NURSING SERVICES, THE NURSING PROCESS IS USED AS THE FRAMEWORK FOR PROVIDING NURSNG CARE TO RECIPIENTS.

*Rationale*

The nursing process (assessment, diagnosis, planning, intervention, and evaluation) enables the nurse to assist the recipient in achieving mutually established goals. Therefore, within organized nursing services each step of the nursing process must be supported.

*Criteria*

1. A nursing information system that includes information on recipient characteristics, nursing diagnoses, the plan of nursing care, interventions, and reports of recipient progress is available.

2. Records used in recording data are accessible to nurses and are maintained in a confidential manner.

3. Record-keeping systems are based on the nursing process; documentation reflects the use of nursing diagnoses.

4. Resources are provided for staff to develop competency in the nursing process, and afford staff the opportunity for validation of nursing diagnoses.

5. Resources are provided for the development of a plan of nursing care derived from nursing diagnoses.

6. There is a mechanism for planning to be recorded, retrieved, and updated.

7. Independent nursing interventions within the scope of nursing practice are encouraged within organized nursing services.

8. Opportunities are provided for nurses to implement the plan of care in collaboration with the recipient, the family, and the interdisciplinary team.

9. A mechanism exists for reviewing and revising staffing patterns (managing human resources) to adequately implement plans of care.

10. Resources are provided to allow the nurse to evaluate care and to develop alternative plans as necessary.

## Standard V. Environment for Practice

AN ENVIRONMENT IS CREATED WITHIN ORGANIZED NURSING SERVICES THAT ENHANCES NURSING PRACTICE AND FACILITATES THE DELIVERY OF CARE BY ALL NURSING STAFF.

*Rationale*

Organized nursing services are in place to provide effective care to recipients. To accomplish this, the practice climate must enable nurses to apply their education and expertise to the fullest extent, and must foster a participative working environment for all nursing staff. This environment promotes the recruitment and retention of qualified, competent nurses.

*Criteria*

1. A written organizational plan exists that is current and delineates lines of authority, accountability, and communication.

2. Collaboration in the planning of care is encouraged within organized nursing services.

3. The nursing staff are oriented to the mission, objectives, and practices of the health care environment; the level of knowledge and skill of the nursing staff is assessed.

4. Resources are provided for participation in educational programs designed to meet the continuing learning needs of nurses for growth and advancement.

5. The performance, educational preparation, and experience of nurses is systematically evaluated and rewarded through recognition and compensation policies.

6. Sufficient support services are in place to facilitate nursing practice.

7. An environment is provided for staff to participate in decision making regarding clinical practice and procedures that affect nursing practice, and clinical issues such as requirements for care, including human and material resources.

8. Roles and responsibilities of practice are consistent with lev-

els of educational preparation and/or competency.

9. Nurse administrators collaborate with the staff of human resources to develop and implement recruitment and retention programs for registered nurses.

10. There is an established system for identifying patient care requirements, allocating nursing resources, and evaluating the system's effectiveness.

## Standard VI. Quality Assurance/Improvement

ORGANIZED NURSING SERVICES HAVE A QUALITY ASSURANCE/IMPROVEMENT PROGRAM.

*Rationale*

Organized nursing services are obligated to provide effective nursing care to society. Standards provide the basis for evaluating care. A quality assurance/improvement program is necessary to determine the degree to which the provision of nursing care complies with standards. A quality assurance/improvement program provides opportunities to improve care and resolve problems.

*Criteria*

1. A written plan exists for the ongoing monitoring and evaluation of nursing care.

2. Nurses participate in the monitoring and evaluation of nursing care in accordance with established professional, regulatory, and organizatonal standards of practice.

3. Actions are taken to resolve problems and improve care; these activities are documented and evaluted for effectiveness.

4. The quality assurance/improvement program itself is periodically evaluated to determine its effectiveness.

5. The quality assurance/improvement program is an integral part of the risk management and quality assurance effort of the organization as a whole.

6. Recipients of nursing care have the opportunity to express their satisfaction and perceptions of the quality of care they have received.

## Standard VII. Ethics

ORGANIZED NURSING SERVICES HAVE POLICIES TO GUIDE ETHICAL DECISION MAKING BASED ON THE *CODE FOR NURSES.*

*Rationale*

Nurses providing care to recipients are confronted with complex ethical dilemmas that require consideration of both the decision-making authority of the recipients and the recipients' requirements for care. The *Code for Nurses* provides the parameters within which the nurse makes ethical judgments.[7]

*Criteria*

1. Nursing is represented in the formal mechanism for resolving ethical dilemmas within the service setting.
2. Educational programs are provided that identify moral, ethical, and legal issues and that support discussions of these issues.
3. Mechanisms are in place for documentaton of self-determination, informed consent, and treatment termination according to applicable laws and regulations.
4. A structure is provided to maintain care within ethical and legal guidelines.
5. Nurses are represented on the health care organizaton's decision-making bodies regarding ethical and legal issues.

## Standard VIII. Research

WITHIN ORGANIZED NURSING SERVICES, RESEARCH IN NURSING, HEALTH, AND NURSING SYSTEMS IS FACILITATED; RESEARCH FINDINGS ARE DISSEMINATED; AND SUPPORT IS PROVIDED FOR INTEGRATION OF THESE FINDINGS INTO THE DELIVERY OF NURSING CARE AND NURSING ADMINISTRATION.

*Rationale*

The continuing advancement of nursing practice and administration depends on the ongoing availability and utilization of a valid and current knowledge base.

*Criteria*

1. Nurses internal and external to organized nursing services are encouraged to conduct both nursing and interdisciplinary research for practice and administration.

2. Opportunities are provided for nurses to gain access to subjects in order to conduct nursing research.

3. A procedure exists for review of proposed research studies, including protection of the rights of human subjects.

4. The dissemination and utilization of nursing research is supported.

## Standard IX. Cultural, Economic, and Social Differences

ORGANIZED NURSING SERVICES PROVIDE POLICIES AND PRACTICES THAT ADDRESS EQUALITY AND CONTINUITY OF NURSING SERVICES, AND THAT RECOGNIZE CULTURAL, ECONOMIC, AND SOCIAL DIFFERENCES AMONG RECIPIENTS SERVED BY THE HEALTH CARE ORGANIZATON.

*Rationale*

Organized nursing services must have policies that promote recognition of cultural, economic, and social differences of recipients and their value systems in order to meet the health care needs of the recipients served.

*Criteria*

1. The policies and practices of organized nursing services reflect the health-related values and traditions of various cultures.

2. Organized nursing services support the nurse advocacy role for all individuals.

3. Planning for and delivery of nursing care incorporate recognition of diverse individual preferences, needs, and capacities for self-care.

4. Mechanisms are provided for nurses and other personnel to identify and discuss their value conflicts.

# LEVELS AND QUALIFICATIONS OF
# NURSE ADMINISTRATORS

Nurse administrators include those nurses who contribute to nursing by directing and coordinating the work of others. For purposes of this discussion, nursing administration has been divided into two administrative levels — those of the nurse executive and the nurse manager — each having a particular focus and making a distinct contribution within a health care organization.

While individual nursing administrative positions may differ from these levels or contain components of more than one level, most nursing administrative positions can be understood within this conceptual schema. How these levels are made operational in a given organization will depend upon the structure and complexity of the organization. Nevertheless, nurse administrators at all levels share a common conceptual framework and use common administrative processes to achieve their goals across all health care settings.

It is the responsibility of the nurse executive and the nurse manager to create a work environment that facilitates and encourages involvement of the staff in decision-making processes. In this way, the nurse closest to the recipients served may make appropriate decisions about care. Creating such an environment may require an adjustment of the administrator's personal leadership style. Communication mechanisms should be in place to facilitate both sending and receiving communication. The integration of the decision-making process, the leadership style(s) of the nursing management team, and communication mechanisms are critical to the accomplishment of the organization's primary goal, which is service to individuals.

Nurses at all levels of the organization expect to participate in decisions affecting their practice. Productivity will be enhanced when nurse administrators promote professional practice and recognize the contributions of nurses.

## Nurse Executive

The nurse executive is responsible for organized nursing services and manages from the perspective of the organization as a whole. While executive management may be shared among several nurse administrators in large health care organizations, this discussion assumes a single nurse executive directing organized nursing services.

As administrators of a significant component of health care organizations, nurse executives exercise the authority inherent in their position to fulfill their responsibility to the organization, the profession, and the health care consumer. They provide leadership and vision for nursing's development and advancement within the organization.

The nurse executive, the spokesperson for organized nursing services, is responsible for the integration of nursing with other functional areas in the mutual achievement of organizational goals. The nurse executive collaborates with other executives in the organization in decision making about health care services and organizational priorities.

As administrator, the nurse executive provides a practice environment that promotes effective and efficient nursing care, an environment that is of primary importance to the recruitment and retention of nurses. Nurse executives ensure the establishment and implementation of standards of nursing practice consistent with standards of professional organizations and regulatory agencies. Nurse executives design systems compatible with nursing standards, the goals of the organization, and changing societal and economic resources. Integral components of the systems design process are cost identification, revenue potential, and impact on the market position of the organization.

Nurse executives have as their primary objective the evaluation of services provided. This is facilitated by ensuring viable quality assurance programs and nursing research activities. Another objective is fostering a climate for practice which enhances productivity and job satisfaction.

Nurse executives assume a leadership role in community and governmental bodies that shape health care policy. They contribute to the development of the health care delivery system, thus providing better health care for society.

The nurse executive, who has primary accountability for the above responsibilities, addresses such responsibilities by collaborating with the nurse manager and the nursing staff to perform the following activities:

1. Participate in the administration of the health care organization.
2. Participate in the strategic and long-range planning of the health care organization.
3. Determine clinical and administrative nursing goals and directions.

4. Determine functions and activities to achieve clinical and administrative goals.
5. Acquire and allocate human, material, and financial resources for specific functions and activities.
6. Evaluate and revise the goals, structures, activities, and resources of organized nursing services.
7. Provide leadership in problem solving.
8. Provide leadership in human resource development and management.
9. Provide opportunities for consumer input into policy development.
10. Ensure the ongoing evaluation of services provided by organized nursing services and the organization as a whole.
11. Facilitate research in the areas of nursing, health, and management systems.
12. Serve as a professional role model to motivate, develop, recruit, and retain future nurse administrators.

The nurse executive is responsible for the management of organized nursing services and accountable for the environment in which clinical nursing is practiced. As a member of executive management, the nurse executive facilitates effective, efficient care of recipients. In providing leadership to nursing, the nurse executive ensures the development, implementation, and evaluation of policies, programs, and services consistent with the organization's mission, goals, and objectives.

## Nurse Manager

The nurse manager is responsible to the nurse executive and manages one or more defined areas of organized nursing services. Nurse managers allocate available resources for efficient and effective nursing care, provide input into executive-level decisions, and keep staff informed of executive-level activities.

Nurse managers coordinate activities between defined areas and provide clinical and administrative leadership and expertise. They facilitate an atmosphere of participative management and the development of collegial relationships among nursing staff. They serve as a link between the nursing staff and other health care disciplines, both within and outside of organized nursing services. Nurse managers have major responsibility for the implementation of the philosophy, goals, and standards of the organization and nursing services within their defined areas of responsibility.

To fulfill the responsibilities described above, nurse managers, in collaboration with the nursing staff, engage in the following activities:

1. Participate in nursing policy formulation and decision making.
2. Accept accountability for services through which direct nursing care is given to recipients.
3. Evaluate the quality and appropriateness of nursing care, including appropriate documentation.
4. Provide guidance for and supervision of personnel accountable to organized nursing services.
5. Coordinate nursing services with the services of other health disciplines.
6. Recruit and select personnel for hire.
7. Staff and schedule personnel.
8. Ensure appropriate orientation, training, and continuing education for personnel.
9. Evaluate performance.
10. Plan and monitor the budget for their defined area.
11. Participate and involve the nursing staff in nursing studies and research.
12. Provide a climate conducive to educational experiences for nursing students.

The nurse manager is accountable for the environment in which clinical nursing is practiced. The ability of the nurse manager to enhance the practice environment is critical to the recruitment and retention of qualified nurses. The manager contributes to the long-range planning process, day-to-day operations, and attainment of goals of the organization. The nurse manager collaborates with the nurse executive and others in organizational programming and committee work.

## Qualifications of Nurse Administrators

Both the nurse executive and the nurse manager must be licensed in the state in which they practice. Beyond licensure, education and experiential qualifications can be identified for individuals functioning at the two levels of nursing administration.

The nurse executive should hold a baccalaureate degree in nursing and a graduate degree in nursing or a related field from a program that includes organizational science and management concepts. Certification by a nationally recognized nursing organization is recommended.

The nurse manager should be prepared with a minimum of a baccalaureate degree in nursing. A master's degree is recommended, as is certification in nursing administration by a nationally recognized nursing organization.

The backgrounds of persons who serve as nurse administrators must include clinical and administrative practice, enabling them to consistently fulfill the responsibilities inherent in the respective administrative roles, which include, but are not limited to, the following:

- Administrative concepts
- Organizational behavior
- Management processes
- Nursing practice standards
- Legal and ethical matters
- Health care economics
- Health and public policy
- Consumer health care issues
- Health care evaluation and outcome measures

It is understood that there are nurse executives and nurse managers who have not attained the qualifications outlined above. It is the intent of this publication to encourage and urge all nurse executives and nurse managers to aspire to and achieve these qualifications.

# APPENDIX
## Comparison of Nurse Administrators' Responsibilities

This appendix differentiates the activities and responsibilities of nurse executives and nurse managers. As noted in the discussion of nursing administrative levels, an administrative position in a given organization may incorporate components of both the nurse executive and nurse manager levels of nursing administration. This appendix, although neither definitive nor all-inclusive, may be of particular assistance to students, nurse educators, and nurses seeking administrative positions.

| Nurse Executive | Nurse Manager |
|---|---|
| 1. Participates in executive-level decision making for the organization. | 1. Particpates in decision-making for organized nursing services. |
| 2. Determines functions within organized nursing services. | 2. Implements functions within a defined area. |
| 3. Conceptualizes and defines the organized nursing services component within the organization. | 3. Interprets and translates the theoretical concepts of nursing into the delivery of nursing services. |
| a. Identifies the philosophy of organized nursing services. | a. Interprets to staff and facilitates the application and implementation of philosophy, objectives, and standards. |
| b. Determines the purpose and objectives of organized nursing services. | b. Interprets specific standards and objectives for a defined area. |
| c. Establishes the nursing care delivery system. | c. Identifies means and monitors achievement of relevant objectives and standards. |

|  Nurse Executive | Nurse Manager |
|---|---|
| d. Ensures that organized nursing services are compatible with requirements of regulatory agencies. | d. Identifies means and monitors compliance with requirements of regulatory agencies. |
| 4. Structures organized nursing services. | 4. Participates in the structuring of organized nursing services. |
| a. Determines defined areas and functions within the structure. | a. Organizes a defined area. |
| b. Describes lines of authority and relationships. | b. Interprets job expectations and lines of authority to staff. |
| c. Determines positions and job specifications. | c. Participates in determining position and job specifications. |
| d. Establishes committees. | d. Assumes leadership roles on committees. |
| 5. Formulates and administers policies and procedures. | 5. Participates in the development or revision of policies and procedures, especially for his or her own operational area. |
| a. Selects policies and procedures that facilitate achievement of organizational goals. | a. Implements policies and procedures in a defined area. |
| b. Integrates nursing policies with organizational policies | b. Integrates policies and practices within a defined area. |
| 6. Determines the management information systems for organized nursing services. | 6. Uses information systems to retrieve, implement, and retain essential records and services. |
| 7. Devises and maintains formal and informal communication systems. | 7. Provides communication liaison between the nurse executive and the staff. |

| Nurse Executive | Nurse Manager |
|---|---|
| 8. Plans for the delivery of nursing and other designated health care services. | 8. Plans, directs, and supervises nursing and health care services for a defined area. |
| a. Selects nursing models. | a. Analyzes nursing care patterns and recommends improvements. |
| b. Plans for evaluation of services. | b. Institutes quality assurance procedures to evaluate the quality of care provided in a defined area. |
| c. Plans for improvement of health care delivery systems. | c. Arranges for continuity of care. |
| d. Establishes mechanisms for ensuring a therapeutic environment for the delivery of services. | d. Collaborates with support services to maintain a safe and therapeutic environment. |
| 9. Identifies needed resources and develops the budget for organized nursing services. | 9. Plans and provides for cost-effective use of resources and participates in budget preparation in a defined area. |
| 10. Ensures that systems are in place to provide for developmental needs of staff and nursing students. | 10. Ensures appropriate orientation and development of staff and nursing students. |
| a. Establishes contractual arrangements with colleges and universities. | a. Identifies learning needs of staff and self. |
| b. Provides for administrative, management, and leadership experiences for students. | b. Schedules learning opportunities for staff. |

| Nurse Executive | Nurse Manager |
|---|---|
| | c. Serves as a role model for staff and students. |
| | d. Provides for clinical experiences for students. |
| 11. Facilitates research in the areas of health, nursing, and management systems. | 11. Participates and involves staff in the research process and the application of findings. |
| 12. Collaborates with appropriate community and governmental policy-making bodies. | 12. Serves as a member or officer of community groups and agencies. |
| 13. Participates and assumes leadership roles in professional organizations and provides opportunities for staff participation. | 13. Participates and assumes leadership roles in professional organizations and encourages staff participation. |

# GLOSSARY

DEFINED AREA. The department or program for which a specific nurse manager has responsibility.

HEALTH CARE ORGANIZATION. The total health care entity within which organized nursing services operate (synonyms for this term include *health care agency* and *institution*).

NURSE ADMINISTRATOR. The nurse who participates in the management of health care services delivery by directing and coordinating the work of nursing and other personnel and representing organized nursing services. The two levels of nursing administration are those of the nurse executive, who is responsible for organized nursing services and manages from the perspective of the organization as a whole, and the nurse manager, who manages one or more defined areas within organized nursing services.

ORGANIZED NURSING SERVICES. The structure through which services are provided by registered nurses under the direction of a nurse executive, within the scope of nursing practice and in accordance with state law.

RECIPIENT OF CARE. The individual provided care by organized nursing services and the family, significant others, and groups of recipients, sometimes including the community (synonyms for this term include *patient, client,* and *consumer*).

STANDARD. A norm that expresses an agreed-upon level of performance that has been developed to characterize, to measure, and to provide guidance for achieving excellence in practice.

# REFERENCES

1. American Hospital Association. 1987. *Report of the Hospital Nursing Personnel Survey 1987.* Chicago: American Hospital Association.

2. American Nurses Association. 1982. *Standards for Organized Nursing Services.* Kansas City, Mo.: American Nurses Association.

3. American Nurses Association. 1978. *Roles, Responsibilities, and Qualifications for Nursing Administrators.* Kansas City, Mo.: American Nurses Association.

4. American Nurses Association. 1973. *Standards of Nursing Practice.* Kansas City, Mo.: American Nurses Association.

5. American Nurses Association. 1980. *Nursing: A Social Policy Statement.* Kansas City, Mo.: American Nurses Association.

6. American Nurses Association. 1985. *Code for Nurses with Interpretive Statements.* Kansas City, Mo.: American Nurses Association.

7. Ibid.

# APPENDIX C
## *Scope and Standards for Nurse Administrators*
## (1995)

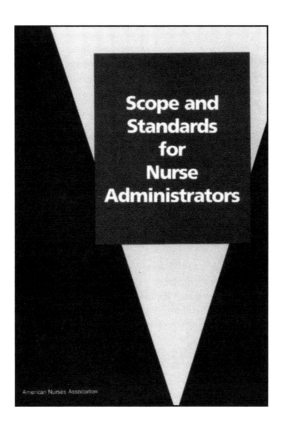

# CONTENTS

# INTRODUCTION

The health care industry, representing one-seventh of the United States economy and being one of its most complex and least predictable service areas, is experiencing a paradigm shift. The goals, stakeholders, services, settings, and types of care are all reconfiguring at a dramatic pace. Competitive forces, societal pressures to hold down costs, and increased demand for access are driving the industry to develop integrated delivery networks, as well as national and regional conglomerates.

The growth of managed care, as an economic strategy to deal with the exponential escalation of health care expenditures, has been a factor in the redesign of the health care delivery system. Shifts in the locus of care are emerging, and will continue to develop. Shifts from episodic care to preventive or restorative care are evidenced by movement from inpatient to outpatient care, increased use of transitional services, increased utilization of home health services, alternative living rather than long-term care, and intensive mental health services. These trends are resulting in closures and downsizing of traditional inpatient care facilities and expansion of community-based services that are creating immediate changes in the management of organized nursing services.

Dramatic demographic changes are impacting the services and settings of health care delivery. These include increasing numbers of frail elderly, immigrants, homeless and indigent persons, and mentally ill. Social changes, such as the spiraling incidence of violence, continuing dissolution of traditional families, the increasing trend for women to work outside the home, and growing needs of rural communities and medically underserved populations, are also shaping health care needs. Within this context there is an increasing focus on legal and ethical issues highlighting greater attention to individual rights.

The reform of health care financing systems is being addressed at the national, state, and community levels. The prospective payment system and capitated systems have given impetus to the development of alternative delivery systems and the increased use of community-based health care. Rapid technological advances have created new educational requirements for health care providers and pose new ethical dilemmas for consumers, policy-makers, and providers. All of these changes bring new challenges and opportunities for nurse administrators across the continuum of care where nursing services are delivered.

The primary goal of organized nursing services is the delivery of quality, compassionate, culturally competent, cost-effective, and efficient nursing care to individuals, families, groups, and communities within the dynamic health care environment. To meet the new demands placed on organized nursing services, nurse administrators must be knowledgeable, skilled, and competent in planning, organizing, leading, and evaluating clinical practice and health care delivery systems.

These standards apply to nurse administrators at all levels across the various settings in which nursing services are delivered.

# SCOPE AND LEVELS OF NURSING ADMINISTRATION PRACTICE, AND QUALIFICATIONS OF NURSE ADMINISTRATORS ACROSS ALL SETTINGS

Nursing administration is conceptually divided into two administrative levels—the nurse executive and the nurse manager—each having a particular focus and making a distinct contribution within a health care system. While individual nursing administrative positions may differ from these levels or contain components of more than one level, most nursing administrative positions can be understood within this conceptual schema. How these levels are made operational in a given organization will depend upon the structure and complexity of the organization. Nevertheless, nurse administrators at all levels share a common conceptual framework and use common administrative processes to achieve their goals across all health care settings.

It is the responsibility of the nurse executive and the nurse manager to create a work environment that facilitates and encourages involvement of the staff in critical thinking to enact professional nursing practice. In this way, the nurse closest to the recipients receiving nursing care may make appropriate decisions. Creating such an environment requires interdisciplinary collaboration and leadership by all nurse administrators. Communication structures and processes need to be in place to facilitate both vertical and horizontal communication. An assessment should be conducted regarding the need for a different management approach for professional and non-professional staff. Broad participation in decision-making processes, leadership style(s) of the nursing management team, and communication systems and processes are critical to the accomplishment of the organization's primary goal, which is service to individuals, families, groups, and communities. Productivity is enhanced when nursing service administrators promote professional practice, recognize the contributions of nurses, and provide appropriate compensation.

**Nurse Executive**

The nurse executive is responsible for organized nursing services and manages from the perspective of the organization as a whole. While executive management responsibilities may be shared among several nurse administrators at differing levels in large health care organizations, and involve people in both line and staff positions, this discussion uses the term nurse executive to refer to all nurse administrators in executive management.

The nurse executive has five primary domains of activity—leading, collaborating, integrating, facilitating, and evaluating. Each domain contributes to the creation and maintenance of environments that develop and support professional nursing practice.

As the administrator of a significant component of health care organizations, the nurse executive exercises the authority inherent in positions to fulfill responsibilities to the profession, the health care consumer, and the organization. The nurse executive provides leadership and vision for nursing's philosophy, development, and advancement within the organization in particular and for society at large. In doing so, the nurse executive is also accountable for the quality and cost-effectiveness of nursing services.

The nurse executive, the chief spokesperson for organized nursing services, is often the catalyst for the integration and collaboration of nursing with other professional disciplines and functional areas in the mutual achievement of client-centered and organizational goals. The nurse executive collaborates with other executives in the organization in making decisions about health care services, settings, and organizational priorities.

As administrator, the nurse executive promotes a practice environment that empowers nurses to provide effective, compassionate, and efficient nursing care. This environment is of primary importance to the recruitment and retention of nurses. Nurse executives identify and implement standards of nursing practice consistent with standards of professional organizations, statutes, and regulations. Nurse executives participate in the design and development of systems compatible with the *ANA Code of Ethics*, nursing standards, the goals and resources of the organization, and changing societal needs and client/family expectations. Integral components of the systems' design process are task and workflow analysis, cost identification, revenue projections, and impact on the market position of the organization.

The nurse executive has another primary objective to evaluate and improve services provided. This is facilitated by ensuring viable quality assessment programs that include nursing research activities. It is also fostered by a climate for practice that enhances job satisfaction through mutual responsibility for productivity and quality improvement.

Nurse executives provide a leadership role in professional, community, and governmental bodies that shape health care policy, thereby contributing to the development of the health care delivery system, and better health care for society.

The nurse executive, who has primary accountability for the above responsibilities, addresses such responsibilities by collaborating with all relevant stakeholders to perform the following activities:

1. Participates in the administration of the health care organization as a full member of the executive team.

2. Participates in the strategic and long-range planning of the health care organization.

3. Provides leadership in the determination of clinical and administrative nursing goals and directions.

4. Participates in the determination of functions and processes to achieve clinical and administrative goals.

5. Acquires and allocates human, material, and financial resources for specific functions and processes.

6. Evaluates and revises the systems and processes of organized nursing services to enhance achievement of identified desired client/family-centered outcomes.

7. Provides leadership in critical thinking, conflict management, and problem solving.

8. Provides leadership in human resource development and management.

9. Provides opportunities for consumer input into personal health care decisions and policy development.

10. Ensures the ongoing evaluation and innovation of services provided by organized nursing services and the organization as a whole.

11. Facilitates the conduct, dissemination, and utilization of research in the areas of nursing, health, and management systems.

12. Serves as a professional role model and mentor to motivate, develop, recruit, and retain future nurse administrators.

13. Serves as a change agent, assisting all staff in understanding the importance, necessity, impact, and process of change.

## Nurse Manager

Nurse managers are responsible to a nurse executive and manage one or more defined areas of organized nursing services. In smaller settings, they may have responsibilities for management of the entire facility and its service. Nurse managers allocate available resources to promote efficient, effective, and compassionate nursing care, provide input into executive-level decisions, and keep staff informed of executive-level activities.

Nurse managers coordinate activities between defined areas, and provide clinical and administrative leadership and expertise. They facilitate an atmosphere of interactive management and the development of collegial relationships among nursing personnel and others. They serve as a link between nursing personnel and other health care disciplines throughout the organizations. Nurse managers have major responsibility for the implementation of the vision, mission, plans, and standards of the organization and nursing services within their defined areas of responsibility.

To fulfill the responsibilities described above, the nurse manager, in collaboration with nursing personnel and members of other disciplines, engages in the following activities:

1. Participates in nursing and organizational policy formulation and decision making.

2. Facilitates participation of staff in nursing and organizational policy formulation and decision making.

3. Accepts organizational accountability for services provided to recipients.

4. Evaluates the quality and appropriateness of care.

5. Provides guidance for and supervision of personnel accountable to the nurse manager.

6. Coordinates nursing services with the services of other health care disciplines.

7. Participates in the recruitment, selection, and retention of personnel.

8. Assumes responsibility for staffing and scheduling personnel. Assignments reflect appropriate utilization of personnel.

9. Assures appropriate orientation, education, credentialing, and continuing professional development for personnel.

10. Evaluates performance of personnel.

11. Participates in planning and monitoring the budget for their defined areas.

12. Participates and involves the nursing staff in evaluative research activities.

13. Fosters a climate conducive to educational experiences for nursing and other students.

14. Fosters peer review.

Nurse managers are accountable for the environment in which clinical nursing is practiced. The ability of nurse managers to enhance the practice environment is critical to the recruitment and retention of nurses with diverse backgrounds and appropriate education and experience. They contribute to the strategic planning process, day-to-day operations, and attainment of goals of the organization. Nurse managers collaborate with the nurse executive and others in organizational planning, innovation, and evaluation.

## Qualifications of Nurse Administrators

Both the nurse executive and the nurse manager must be licensed in the state in which they practice. Beyond licensure, education and experiential qualifications can be identified for professional nurses functioning at the two levels of nursing administration.

The nurse executive should hold a baccalaureate degree in nursing and a graduate degree in nursing, or a related field, from a program that includes organizational science and management concepts, or demonstrate equivalent competencies. The nurse executive should also hold certification in nursing administration by a nationally recognized nursing organization.

The nurse manager should be prepared with a minimum of a baccalaureate degree in nursing, or a baccalaureate in a related field, or demonstrate equivalent competencies. A master's degree is recommended, as is certification in nursing administration by a nationally recognized nursing organization.

The backgrounds of professional nurses who serve as nurse administrators must include clinical and administrative practice, which enables nurses to consistently fulfill the responsibilities inherent in the respective administrative roles. The nurse administrator's practice draws on knowledge and research from the following areas:

Organizational behavior

Management systems and processes

Nursing practice standards

Clinical practice guidelines

Law, regulation, and ethics

Health care economics

Health and public policy

Trends in business practices

Consumer health care issues

Health care evaluation and outcome measures

Fiscal management and finance

It is understood that there are nurse executives and nurse managers who have not attained these qualifications. It is the intent of this publication to encourage and urge all nurse executives and nurse managers to aspire to and achieve these qualifications.

# STANDARDS OF CARE

**Standard I. Assessment**

**The nurse administrator develops, maintains, and evaluates patient/client and staff data collection systems and processes to support the practice of nursing and delivery of patient care.**

*Measurement Criteria*

The nurse administrator:

1. Identifies assessment elements including nursing-sensitive indicators appropriate to a given organizational context.
2. Utilizes current research findings and current practice guidelines and standards to modify data collection elements.
3. Monitors and evaluates assessment processes that are sensitive to the unique and diverse needs of individuals and target populations.
4. Identifies and documents the necessary resources to support data collection, and advocates for appropriate resources.
5. Analyzes the workflow related to effectiveness and efficiency of assessment processes in the target environment.
6. Develops, maintains, and evaluates systems for efficient data collection as part of the overall institutional data collection system.
7. Promotes, maintains, and evaluates a data collection system in an accessible and retrievable format.
8. Initiates processes to modify information systems as needed to meet changing data requirements and needs.
9. Devises criteria and establishes procedures to assure confidentiality of data.
10. Facilitates integration of unified assessment processes developed in collaboration with other health care disciplines and across the continuum of care.

11. Evaluates assessment practices to assure timely, reliable, valid, and comprehensive data collection.

12. Works in conjunction with appropriate departments.

## Standard II. Diagnosis

**The nurse administrator develops, maintains, and evaluates an environment that supports the professional nurse in analysis of assessment data and in decisions to determine relevant diagnoses.**

*Measurement Criteria*

The nurse administrator:

1. Identifies and advocates for adequate resources for decision analysis in conjunction with appropriate departments.

2. Assists and supports staff in developing and maintaining competency in the diagnostic process.

3. Facilitates interdisciplinary collaboration in data analysis and decision-making processes.

4. Promotes an organizational climate that supports validation of diagnoses.

5. Develops, maintains, and evaluates a format for documentation of diagnoses that facilitates development of a client-centered plan of care and determination of desired outcomes.

## Standard III. Identification of Outcomes

**The nurse administrator develops, maintains, and evaluates information processes that promote desired, client-centered outcomes.**

*Measurement Criteria*

The nurse administrator:

1. Participates in the design and development of multidisciplinary processes to establish and maintain standards consistent with the identified client-centered outcomes.

2. Facilitates nurse and other staff member participation in interdisciplinary identification of desired client-centered outcomes.

3. Assists in identification, development, and utilization of databases that include nursing-sensitive measures and desired client-centered outcomes.

4. Facilitates nurse participation in the monitoring and evaluation of nursing care in accordance with established professional, regulatory, and organizational standards of practice.

5. Promotes the integration of clinical, human resource, and financial data to support decision making.

6. Fosters establishment and continuous improvement of clinical guidelines linked to client outcomes that provide direction for continuity of care, and are attainable with available resources.

7. Works in conjunction with appropriate departments.

## Standard IV. Planning

**The nurse administrator develops, maintains, and evaluates organizational planning systems to facilitate the delivery of nursing care.**

*Measurement Criteria*

The nurse administrator:

1. Contributes to the development and continuous improvement of organizational systems in which plans related to the delivery of nursing services can be developed, modified, documented, and evaluated.

2. Contributes to the development and continuous improvement of organizational systems that support prioritization of activities within plans related to the delivery of nursing services and patient care.

3. Contributes to the development and continuous improvement of mechanisms for plans to be recorded, retrieved, and updated across the continuum of care.

4. Advocates organizational processes that allow for creativity in the development of alternative plans for achieving desired, client-centered, cost-effective outcomes.

5. Fosters interdisciplinary planning and collaboration that focuses on the individuals and populations served.

6. Promotes the integration of applicable contemporary management and organizational theories, nursing and related research findings, and practice standards and guidelines into the planning process.

7. Assists and supports staff in developing and maintaining competency in the planning and change process.

8. Advocates integration of policies into action plans for achieving desired client-centered outcomes.

9. Participates in the development, implementation, and use of a system for preventing and reporting abuse of client's rights, and incompetent, unethical, or illegal practices by health care providers.

10. Reviews and evaluates plans for appropriate utilization of staff at all levels of practice in accordance with the provision of the state's nurse practice act and the professional standards of practice.

11. Integrates clinical, human resource, and financial data to appropriately plan standards of nursing and patient care, facilitating continuity across a continuum.

12. Works in conjunction with appropriate departments.

## Standard V. Implementation

**The nurse administrator develops, maintains, and evaluates organizational systems that support implementation of the plan.**

*Measurement Criteria*

The nurse administrator:

1. Participates in the development, evaluation, and maintenance of organizational systems that integrate policies and procedures with regulations, practice standards, and clinical guidelines.

2. Collaborates in the design and improvement of systems and the identification of resources that support interventions that are consistent with the established plans.

3. Collaborates in the design and improvement of systems and the identification of resources that assure interventions are safe, effective, efficient, and culturally competent.

4. Collaborates in the design and improvement of systems and processes that assure interventions are implemented by the most appropriate personnel.

5. Collaborates in the design and improvement of systems to assure appropriate and efficient documentation of interventions.

6. Facilitates staff participation in decision making regarding the development and implementation of organizational systems, and the specification of resources necessary for implementation of the plan.

7. Works in conjunction with appropriate departments.

### Standard VI. Evaluation

**The nurse administrator evaluates the plan and its progress in relation to the attainment of outcomes.**

*Measurement Criteria*

The nurse administrator:

1. Promotes implementation of processes and resources that deliver data and information to empower staff to participate meaningfully in clinical decision making.

2. Advocates for educational opportunities for staff specific to current interventions, available technologies, or other skills to enhance ability to promote quality in health care delivery.

3. Utilizes appropriate research methods and findings to improve care processes, structures, and measurement of client-centered outcomes.

4. Facilitates the participation of staff in the systematic, interdisciplinary, and ongoing evaluation of programs, processes, and desired client-centered outcomes.

5. Sets priorities for allocation of resources.

6. Advocates for resources sufficient to provide time for critical assessment and evaluation of desired client-centered outcomes.

7. Fosters participation and recognition of staff in formal and informal organizational committees, teams, and task forces.

8. Advocates for and supports a process of governance that includes participation of nurses.

9. Participates in the peer review and privileging process for advanced practice nurses.

10. Supports effective information-handling processes and technologies that facilitate evaluation of effectiveness and efficiency of decisions, plans, and activities in relation to desired client-centered outcomes.

11. Promotes the development of policies, procedures, and guidelines based on research findings and institutional measurement of quality outcomes.

12. Utilizes data generated from outcome research to develop innovative changes in patient care delivery.

# STANDARDS OF PROFESSIONAL PERFORMANCE

## Standard I. Quality of Care and Administrative Practice

**The nurse administrator systematically evaluates the quality and effectiveness of nursing practice and nursing services administration.**

*Measurement Criteria*

The nurse administrator:

1. Identifies key quality indicators for monitoring and evaluating.
2. Analyzes data and information to identify opportunities for improving services, using appropriate internal and external data.
3. Develops, implements, and evaluates systems and processes that complement the overall system for performance improvement.
4. Participates in interdisciplinary evaluation teams.

## Standard II. Performance Appraisal

**The nurse administrator evaluates her/his own performance based on professional practice standards, relevant statutes and regulations, and organizational criteria.**

*Measurement Criteria*

The nurse administrator:

1. Engages in self-performance appraisal on a regular basis, identifying areas of strength as well as areas for professional/practice development.
2. Seeks constructive feedback regarding her/his own practice.

3. Takes action to achieve goals identified during performance appraisal.

4. Participates in peer review as appropriate.

## Standard III. Education

**The nurse administrator acquires and maintains current knowledge in administrative practice.**

*Measurement Criteria*

The nurse administrator:

1. Seeks additional knowledge and skills appropriate to the practice setting by developing and/or participating in educational programs and activities, conferences, workshops, interdisciplinary professional meetings, and self-directed learning.

2. Seeks experiences to expand and maintain skills and knowledge base.

3. Gains appropriate formal education and/or certification for career path.

4. Networks with peers in state/region to share ideas and conduct mutual problem solving.

## Standard IV. Collegiality

**The nurse administrator fosters a professional environment.**

*Measurement Criteria*

The nurse administrator:

1. Promotes understanding and effective use of organization, management, and nursing theories and research.

2. Contributes to nursing management education and professional development of staff, students, and colleagues.

3. Shares knowledge and skills with colleagues and others, and acts as a role model/mentor.

4. Creates a climate of effective communication.

5. Contributes to an environment of mutual respect and understanding.

## Standard V. Ethics

**The nurse administrator's decisions and actions are based on ethical principles.**

*Measurement Criteria*

The nurse administrator:

1. Advocates on behalf of recipients of services and personnel.
2. Maintains privacy, confidentiality, and security of patient, client, staff, and organization data.
3. Advocates organizational adherence to the *ANA Code for Nurses*.
4. Fosters a non-discriminatory climate in which care is delivered in a manner sensitive to sociocultural diversity.
5. Supports the system to address ethical issues within nursing and the organization.

## Standard VI. Collaboration

**The nurse administrator collaborates with nursing staff at all levels, interdisciplinary teams, executive officers, and other stakeholders.**

*Measurement Criteria*

The nurse administrator:

1. Facilitates collaboration within organized nursing services and the organization.
2. Collaborates with nursing staff and other disciplines at all levels in the development, implementation, and evaluation of programs and services.
3. Collaborates with administrative peers in determining the acquisition, allocation, and utilization of organizational fiscal and human resources.

4. Collaborates with the human resources staff to develop and implement recruitment and retention programs for staff.

5. Provides the opportunity for ongoing communication between self and staff.

6. Collaborates with other providers of nursing/patient care within the delivery system for provision of seamless delivery of services.

## Standard VII. Research

**The nurse administrator supports research and integrates it into the delivery of nursing care and nursing administration.**

*Measurement Criteria*

The nurse administrator:

1. Fosters the identification of areas suitable for nursing research.

2. Supports procedures for review of proposed research studies, including protection of the rights of human subjects.

3. Facilitates the conduct and utilization of research and other scholarly activities.

4. Advocates for resources to support research.

5. Promotes research based on knowledge-driven nursing practice.

## Standard VIII. Resource Utilization

**The nurse administrator evaluates and administers the resources of organized nursing services.**

*Measurement Criteria*

The nurse administrator:

1. Evaluates factors related to safety, outcomes, effectiveness, cost, and social impact when developing and implementing practice innovations.

2. Delegates responsibilities appropriate to the licensure, education, and experience of staff.

3. Evaluates and maintains management information systems that provide integrated data needed to monitor and explain variances from established parameters.

4. Designs and negotiates organizational acceptance of appropriate roles for the utilization of all staff.

5. Negotiates for appropriate role expansion and delimitation.

6. Monitors and evaluates appropriate utilization of staff.

7. Advocates to secure appropriate fiscal and human resources to accomplish the work/goals of the service.

# GLOSSARY

| | |
|---|---|
| **Client-centered care** | Therapeutics delivered to provide coordinated continuity among services that is congruent with patient- and family-desired outcomes. |
| **Continuity of care** | An interdisciplinary process that includes clients and significant others in the development and implementation of a plan of coordinated care. This process facilitates the client's transition between settings, based on changing needs and available resources. |
| **Criteria** | Relevant, measurable indicators of the standards of clinical nursing practice. |
| **Cultural competence** | A complex integration of knowledge, attitudes, and skills that enhances cross-cultural communication and appropriate/effective interactions with others. |
| **Defined area** | The department or program for which a specific nurse manager has responsibility. |
| **Develops** | Refers to the process of analyzing, designing, modifying, and implementing a coordinated plan of care. |
| **Education** | Refers to knowledge and cognitive development. |
| **Executive** | The person or body in whom the supreme, or highest, executive power is vested. |

| | |
|---|---|
| **Guidelines** | Describe a process of client care management that has the potential to improve the quality of clinical and consumer decision making. Guidelines are systematically developed statements based on available scientific evidence and expert opinion. |
| **Health care organization** | The total health care entity within which organized nursing services operate (synonyms for this term include health care agency and institution). |
| **Interdisciplinary** | Characterized by full participation and/or cooperation of two or more people from different disciplines or fields of study in a task. |
| **Leading** | An activity that involves change, innovation, growth, and empowerment of self and others. |
| **Nurse** | Refers to registered nurses at all levels in the organization. |
| **Nurse administrator** | The nurse whose primary function is the management of health care services delivery, and who represents organized nursing services. The two levels of nursing administration are those of the nurse executive and the nurse manager. |
| **Nurse executive** | The nurse who is responsible for organized nursing services and manages from the perspective of the organization as a whole. Her/his five primary domains of activity are leading, collaborating, facilitating, integrating, and evaluating. |

| | |
|---|---|
| **Nurse manager** | The nurse who manages one or more defined areas within organized nursing services. Her/his primary domains of activity are planning, organizing, leading, and evaluating. |
| **Nursing** | The diagnosis and treatment of human responses to actual or potential health problems. |
| **Nursing sensitive** | Measures and indicators that reflect the impact of nursing actions on outcomes. |
| **Organized nursing services** | The structure through which services are provided by registered nurses and other personnel under the direction of a nurse administrator, within the scope of nursing practice, and in accordance with state law. |
| **Plan** | A process of establishing and prioritizing activities for clients, management, financial/business, and program goals. |
| **Recipient of care** | The individual, family, group, or community provided care by organized nursing services (synonyms for this term include patient, client, and consumer). |
| **Staff** | Refers to all personnel reporting to the nurse administrator. |
| **Stakeholders** | Refers to all parties with a vested interest in, or who would be significantly impacted by, the outcomes of a particular situation, program, or activity (i.e., nursing staff at all levels, interdisciplinary teams, executive officers, and third party payers). |

| | |
|---|---|
| **Standard** | Authoritative statement enunciated and promulgated by the profession by which the quality of practice, service, or education can be judged. |
| **Standards of care** | Authoritative statements that describe a competent level of clinical nursing practice demonstrated through assessment, diagnosis, outcome identification, planning, implementation, and evaluation. |
| **Standards of nursing practice** | Authoritative statements that describe a level of care or performance common to the profession of nursing by which the quality of nursing practice can be judged. Standards of clinical nursing practice include both standards of care and standards of professional performance. |
| **Standards of professional performance** | Authoritative statements that describe a competent level of behavior in the professional role, including activities related to quality of care, performance appraisal, education, collegiality, ethics, collaboration, research, and resource utilization. |
| **Target population** | The identified individuals, family, group, or community to be recipients of care. |
| **Training** | Refers to skill development education. |

# REFERENCES

1. American Nurses Association. 1991. *Standards for Organized Nursing Services, and Responsibilities of Nurse Administrators Across All Settings.* Kansas City, Mo.: American Nurses Association.

2. ___. 1991. *Standards of Clinical Nursing Practice.* Kansas City, Mo.: American Nurses Association.

3. ___. 1995. *Standards of Practice for Nursing Informatics.* Washington, D.C.: American Nurses Association.

4. ___. 1985. *Code for Nurses with Interpretive Statements.* Washington, D.C.: American Nurses Association.

5. ___. 1995. *Nursing's Social Policy Statement.* Washington, D.C.: American Nurses Association.

6. Barker, A. 1992. *Transformational Nursing Leadership.* Baltimore, Md.: Williams and Wilkins.

7. Koerner, JoEllen G., and Karpiuk, K.L. 1994. *Implementing Differential Nursing Practice.* Gaithersburg, Md.: Aspen.

# INDEX

*Note:* Entries designated with a calendar year in brackets indicates an entry from an earlier edition or predecessor publication. [1991] is *Standards for Organized Nursing Services and Responsibilities of Nurse Administrators across All Settings.* [1995] is the first edition *Scope and Standards for Nurse Administrators.*

## A

Accountability, 4, 5
    nurse manager and, 8, 9
    professional environment and, 26
    [1991], 41, 45
Advocacy
    ethics and, 27
    evaluation and, 21
    nurse manager and, 7, 9
    planning and, 18, 19
    professional environment and, 26
    quality of care and, 23
    research and, 29
    rights and, 35
    [1991], 43, 48
    [1995], 71, 72, 74, 79, 80, 81
Age-appropriate care. *See* Cultural
    competence
American Nurses Association (ANA)
    Committee on Nursing Practice
        Standards and Guidelines, *v*
    Congress of Nursing Practice, *v*
    [1991], 40
American Nurses Credentialing
    Center (ANCC), *v*
American Organization of Nurse
    Executives (AONE), *v*
Analysis. *See* Critical thinking,
    analysis, and synthesis
Assessment
    evaluation and, 21
    standard of care [1995], 71–72
    standard of practice, 15
    [1991], 44
Association of State and Territorial
    Directors of Nursing (ASTDN), *v*

Autonomy, 3, 4
    professional environment and, 26

## B

*Bill of Rights for Registered Nurses*
    (2001), 26, 35

## C

Case management. *See* Coordination
    of care
Certification and credentialing
    evaluation and, 21
    nurse administrator and, 11
        [1991], 42
    nurse manager and, 9
    professional knowledge and, 25
    resource utilization and, 30
    [1995], 78, 81
Client. *See* Patient
Client-centered care (defined)
    [1995], 82
*Code of Ethics for Nurses with*
    *Interpretive Statements*, 27, 35
    [1991], 41
    [1995], 66, 79
    *See also* Ethics
Collaboration
    assessment and, 15
    implementation and, 20
    outcome identification and, 17
    nurse executive and, 5
    nurse manager and, 8
    planning and, 19
    standard of professional
        performance, 28
    [1995], 79-80

Collaboration *(Cont.)*
    [1991], 42, 45, 46
    [1995], 65, 71, 72, 73, 74, 75, 80
    *See also* Interdisciplinary
      healthcare teams
Collegiality, 2, 7
    standard of professional
      performance [1995], 78
Communication
    importance of, 4
    professional environment and, 26
    research and, 29
    [1991], 45, 48
    [1995], 65, 78, 80
Community health care, 3
    collaboration and, 28
    *See also* Practice settings
Compensation. *See under* Human
  resources
Competency
    diagnosis and, 16
    nurse executive and, 5
    nurse manager and, 9
    performance appraisal and, 24
    planning and, 18
    [1991], 44, 46
    [1995], 72, 74
Competence assessment. *See*
  Certification and credentialing
Confidentiality, 1, 2
    assessment and, 15
    ethics and, 27
    [1991], 44
    [1995], 71, 79
Consultation, 3
Consumer needs, 1, 6, 23
Continuity of care
    defined, 31
      [1995], 82
    demand for, 1
    outcome identification and, 17
    [1995], 73, 74

Continuum of care, 5, 8, 15, 18, 19, 20, 30
Coordination of care
    facilitation of, 1
    nurse manager and, 7, 8
    *See also* Interdisciplinary
      healthcare teams
Core ideology of nursing
    defined, 31
    nurse executive and, 5
    professional environment and, 26
Cost control, 2, 3, 5
    nurse manager and, 8, 9
    planning and, 18, 19
    quality of care and, 23
    resource utilization and, 30
    [1991], 43
    [1995], 73, 74, 80
Cost-effectiveness. *See* Cost control
Credentialing. *See* Certification and
  credentialing
Criteria
    assessment, 15
    collaboration, 28
    defined, 31
      [1995], 82
    diagnosis, 16
    ethics, 27
    implementation, 20
    outcome identification, 17
    performance appraisal, 24
    planning, 18–19
    professional environment, 26
    professional knowledge, 25
    quality of care and administrative
      practice, 23
    research, 29
    resource utilization, 30
Critical thinking, analysis, and
  synthesis, 3, 6
    assessment and, 15
    diagnosis and, 16
    work environment and, 4

[1995], 65
[1995], 71, 72
Culture. *See under* Nursing
Cultural competence, 6, 7
    assessment and, 15
    defined [1995], 82
    ethics and, 27
    implementation and, 20
    nurse manager and, 8
    [1995], 71, 75, 79
Cultural, economic, and social
  differences
    standard for nursing services
      [1991], 48

**D**
Data collection, 5
    assessment and, 15
    defined, 31
    study program (NDNQI), 7
    [1995], 71, 72
Decision-making
    diagnosis and, 16
    evaluation and, 21
    implementation and, 20
    leadership and, 2
    nurse administrator and [1991], 43
    nurse manager and, 7, 8
    outcome identification and, 17
    planning and, 19
    professional environment and, 26
    work environment and, 4
    [1995], 65, 72, 73, 75
Defined area (defined)
    [1991], 58
    [1995], 82
Develops (defined) [1995], 82
Delivery systems. *See* Healthcare
delivery systems; Nursing care
delivery systems
Diagnosis
    standard of care [1995], 72

standard of practice, 16
    [1991], 44
Documentation
    diagnosis and, 16
    implementation and, 20
    planning and, 18
    quality of care and, 23
    [1991], 41, 44, 45, 46, 47
    [1995], 72, 73, 75

**E**
Economic issues. *See* Cost control
Education
    defined [1995], 82
    implementation and, 21
    importance of, 1, 4
    nurse administrator and, 11
    nurse executive and, 5
    nurse manager and, 9
    professional environment and, 26
    professional knowledge and, 25
    resource utilization and, 30
    standard of professional
      performance [1995], 78
    [1991], 45, 46, 47
    [1995], 75, 78, 81
Empowerment, 4, 21
    [1995], 75
Environment for practice
    standard for nursing services
      [1991], 45–46
Ethics, 3
    code, 27, 35
      [1991], 41
      [1995], 66, 79
    nurse executive and, 6
    nurse manager and, 8
    planning and, 18
    research and, 2, 29
    standard for nursing services
      [1991], 47

Ethics *(Cont.)*
    standard of professional
        performance, 27
        [1995], 79
        [1995], 74, 80
Evaluation, 3, 6
    collaboration and, 28
    outcome identification and, 17
    planning and, 18
    resource utilization and, 30
    standard of care [1995], 75–76
    standard of practice, 21
    [1991], 44, 45, 46
    [1995], 72, 73, 77, 79
Evidence-based practice, 4, 6, 7
    defined, 31
    nurse manager and, 8, 9
    professional environment and, 26
    [1995], 80
    *See also* Research
Executive (defined) [1995], 82

**F**
Financial issues. *See* Cost control
Fiscal resource management
    standard for nursing services
        [1991], 43

**G**
Guidelines, 15, 17, 18, 20, 21, 29
    (defined) [1995], 83

**H**
Healthcare delivery systems, 5, 6, 7, 11
Healthcare environment, 1–2
Healthcare organization (defined), 31
    [1991], 58
    [1995], 83
Healthcare policy, 5
    nurse executive and, 5
    nurse manager and, 8
    [1991], 42–43, 48

Healthcare providers
    evaluation and, 21
    information sharing by, 2
    *See also* Interdisciplinary
        healthcare teams
Hospice and Palliative Nurses
    Association (HPNA), *v*
Human resources, 3, 6
    collaboration and, 28
    collective bargaining, 35
    compensation, 4, 35
        [1995], 65
    leadership and, 2
    nurse manager and, 9
    planning and, 19
    resource utilization and, 30
    [1991], 44
    [1995], 73, 74, 79, 80, 81
    *See also* Professional
        development; Recruitment
        and retention

**I**
Implementation
    standard of care [1995], 74–75
    standard of practice, 20
Information systems
    assessment and, 15
    evaluation and, 21
    outcome identification and, 17
    sharing, 2
    [1991], 43, 44
    [1995], 71, 73, 81
Integration of systems, 2
    [1995], 73
Intellectual capital
    defined, 31
    resource utilization and, 30
Interdisciplinary (defined) [1995], 83
Interdisciplinary healthcare
    assessment and, 15
    diagnosis and, 16

Nurse administrator *(Cont.)*
    responsibilities, 4
        [1991], 49
        [1995], 65–69
    roles, 3
    standard for nursing services
        [1991], 42–43
    *See also* Nurse executive; Nurse
        manager; Standards of
        practice; Standards of
        professional performance
Nurse executive, 4
    activities, 6–7
        [1991], 50–51
        [1995], 67–68
    alternative titles, 7
    authority, 11
    compared to nurse manager,
        10–11
        [1991], 54–57
    defined, 5, 31
        [1991], 42
        [1995], 65, 83
    responsibilities, 5–7, 11
        [1991], 49–51
        [1995], 66–67
Nurse manager, 4
    activities, 8–9
        [1991], 52
        [1995], 68–69
    alternative titles, 9
    authority, 11
    compared to nurse executive,
        10–11
        [1991], 54–57
    defined, 7, 31
        [1991], 42
        [1995], 65, 84
    resource utilization, 7
    responsibilities, 7–9, 11
        [1991], 51–52
        [1995], 68, 69

Nurse-sensitive (defined), 31
    [1995], 84
Nursing
    culture, 1
    defined [1995], 84
    obligation to society, 35
    performance appraisal and, 24
    quality of care and, 23
    services (defined), 32
    shortage, 1
    work environment, 4, 35
    *See also* Education; Registered
        Nurse
*Nursing: A Social Policy Statement*
    (1980) [1991], 41
Nursing Advisory Council on Nurse
    Education and Practice, 7
Nursing care delivery systems, 6
Nursing models, 2, 23
Nursing process, 13
    standard for nursing services
        [1991], 44
Nursing services. *See* Organized
    nursing services
*Nursing's Agenda for the Future*
    (2002), 6

**O**
Organized nursing services (defined)
    [1991], 58
    [1995], 84
Outcomes, 5, 7
    diagnosis and, 16
    evaluation and, 21
    planning and, 18, 19
    quality of care and, 23
    research and, 29
    resource utilization and, 30
    standard of care for identifying
        [1995], 72–73
    standard of practice for
        identifying, 17
        [1995], 74, 80

**P**

Patient
    defined, 32
    outcome identification and, 17
    planning and, 18
    resource utilization and, 30
    [1991], 44, 46, 48
Peer review
    performance appraisal and, 24
    [1995], 77, 78
Performance appraisal
    nurse manager and, 9
    standard of professional
      performance, 24
        [1995], 77–78
    [1991], 45
Patient care delivery systems, 5, 6, 7, 11
Patient care planning. *See* Planning
Personnel. *See* Human resources
Philosophy and structure
    standard for nursing services
      [1991], 41
Plan (defined) [1995], 84
Planning
    diagnosis and, 16
    evaluation and, 21
    implementation and, 20
    performance appraisal and, 24
    research and, 29
    standard of care [1995], 73–74
    standard of practice, 18–19
    strategic, 3, 8
    [1991], 44, 45, 46, 48
    [1995], 75
Policy. *See* Healthcare policy
Practice levels. *See* Nurse
  administrator, levels of practice
Practice settings, 1, 3
Preceptors. *See* Mentoring
Privacy. *See* Confidentiality
Problem identification. *See* Diagnosis

Problem-solving
    professional knowledge and, 25
    [1995], 78
Professional development, 3, 5
    evaluation and, 21
    leadership and, 2
    nurse manager and, 9
    performance appraisal and, 24
    professional environment and, 26
    professional knowledge and, 25
    quality of care and, 23
    [1991], 41
    [1995], 77
    *See also* Education; Human
      resources; Leadership
Professional environment
    standard of professional
      performance, 26
Professional knowledge
    standard of professional
      performance, 25
    *See also* Education
Professional performance
    *See* Standards of professional
      performance

**Q**

Quality assurance/improvement
    standard for nursing services
      [1991], 46
Quality of care, 3, 4
    nurse manager and, 8
    [1995], 73, 75, 77
Quality of care and administrative
  practice
    collaboration and, 28
    evaluation and, 21
    resource utilization and, 30
    standard of professional
      performance, 23
      [1995], 77

**R**

Recipient of care (defined)
    [1991], 58
    [1995], 84
Recruitment and retention, 5
    nurse manager and, 8
    professional environment and, 26
    [1991], 46
    [1995], 80
    *See also* Human resources
Registered nurse (RN)
    autonomy, 3, 4, 5
    bill of rights, 26, 35
    decision-making and, 6, 7
    outcome identification and, 17
    professional trends, 1
    recruitment and retention, 5, 8
    *See also* Nursing
Regulatory issues. *See* Laws, statutes,
  and regulations
Reimbursement, 1
Research, 3, 4, 6
    assessment and, 15
    evaluation and, 21
    nurse executive and, 5, 6
    nurse manager and, 9
    planning and, 18
    professional environment and, 26
    standard for nursing services
      [1991], 47
    standard of professional
      performance, 29
        [1995], 80
    [1995], 71, 74, 75, 78
    *See also* Evidence-based practice
Resource utilization, 2
    assessment and, 15
    diagnosis and, 16
    evaluation and, 21
    implementation and, 20
    nurse executive and, 6, 7
    nurse manager and, 7

outcome identification and, 17
planning and, 18
research and, 29
standard of professional
    performance, 30
      [1995], 80–81
  [1991], 45
  [1995], 71, 72, 75, 79, 81
*Roles, Responsibilities, and*
  *Qualifications for Nurse*
  *Administrators* (1978) [1991], 40

**S**

Safety assurance, 4, 7, 35
    quality of care and, 23
    resource utilization and, 30
    [1995], 75, 80
Scope of practice, 3–11
    development, 1
    nurse manager, 9
    [1995], 65–69
*Scope and Standards for Nurse*
  *Administrators* (1995), v, 61–84
Settings. *See* Practice settings
Scientific findings. *See* Research;
  Evidence-based practice
Spiritual issues
    *See* Cultural competence
Staff
    defined, 32
    empowerment, 20, 21
    [1995], 84
    *See also* Human resources
Stakeholders (defined) [1995], 84
Standards, 7
    defined, 13, 32
      [1991], 58
Standards for organized nursing
  services [1991], 41–48
    cultural, economic, and social
      differences, 48
    environment for practice, 45–46

**V**

Values
    nurse executive and, 5
    nurse manager and, 8
    professional environment and, 26
    [1991], 45, 48

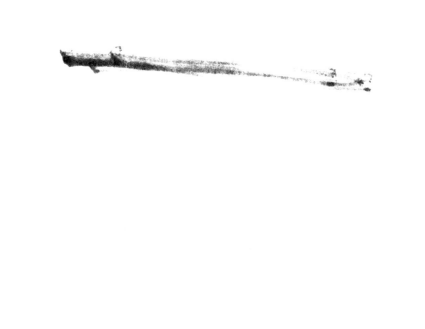

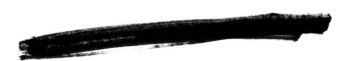